Changing and Learning in the Lives of Physicians

Changing and Learning in the Lives of Physicians

EDITED BY

Robert D. Fox
Paul E. Mazmanian
R. Wayne Putnam

FOREWORD BY MALCOLM S. KNOWLES

PRAEGER

New York
Westport, Connecticut
London

Library of Congress Cataloging-in-Publication Data

Changing and learning in the lives of physicians / [edited by] Robert
D. Fox, Paul E. Mazmanian, R. Wayne Putnam.
    p.   cm.
  Bibliography: p.
  Includes index.
  Contents: An overview / Robert D. Fox, Paul E. Mazmanian, R. Wayne
Putnam — Curiosity / Salvatore S. Lanzilotti — Personal well-being
/ Patricia Iverson, Robert D. Fox — Financial well-being / Richard
Caplan, Harry Gallis — Age and stage of career development / Nancy
L. Bennett, Martin O. Hotvedt — Sense of professional competency /
R. Wayne Putnam, M. Donald Campbell — The clinical environment /
David Davis — Medical institutions / Jocelyn M. Lockyer, John
Parboosingh — Professional peers / Harold Paul, Charles Osborne —
Regulations / Paul E. Mazmanian, Peter O. Fried — Family and
community roles / Jacqueline Parochka, Robert D. Fox — A theory of
change and learning / Robert D. Fox, Paul Mazmanian, and R. Wayne
Putnam.
  ISBN 0–275–93338–5 (alk. paper)
  1. Physicians.   2. Medical education.   3. Medical innovations.
4. Continuing education.   I. Fox, Robert D.   II. Mazmanian, Paul E.
III. Putnam, R. Wayne.
  R690.C42   1989
  610.69—dc20   89–3886

Library of Congress Catalog Card Number: 89–3886
ISBN: 0–275–93338–5

First published in 1989

Praeger Publishers, One Madison Avenue, New York, NY 10010
A division of Greenwood Press, Inc.

Printed in the United States of America

The paper used in this book complies with the
Permanent Paper Standard issued by the National
Information Standards Organization (Z39.48–1984).

10 9 8 7 6 5 4 3 2 1

Foreword

This volume makes at least four unique contributions to the literature of adult education in general, and continuing medical education in particular:

1. It provides a vast array of descriptions of techniques and resources that continuing learners have found to be useful.
2. It models a qualitative approach to social science research that offers a much more productive way of discovering the important variables in the processes and dynamics of lifelong learning than the traditional quantitative and correlational approaches—but at the same time lays a rich foundation of potential hypotheses for subsequent empirical research.
3. It offers the beginning of a theoretical framework for conceptualizing the phenomena of continuing education that serves as a guide for practical experimentation and further development of theory.
4. It presents continuing education as a highly human, personal, and creative enterprise in contrast to the more institutionalized, prescriptive, and mechanistic undertaking, as it so often has been depicted.

This volume generates several strong impressions. One of the sharpest impressions that it gives us is a cumulative documentation of the fact that the medical profession is well into an era of accelerating technological and conceptual change. This makes continuing medical education not only a desirable, but an essential societal imperative—and if this is true of medicine, think of all the other professions and occupations of which it is equally true. A second strong impression is that it looked at its continuing learners as whole people, not just as narrow practitioners of a profession. A third impression is that it begins to portray continuing medical education as a system of learners with needs to change, and a system of multiple resources—material, human, and environmental—for helping them meet those needs. It makes it clear that the present linking of these resources with learners' needs is haphazard and fragmentary, and that one of the critical challenges of the decades ahead is to conceptualize and operationalize the continuing education enterprise as a system of learning resources for use by learners in self-planned projects of continuing personal and professional development.

A final impression is that Robert Fox and his collaborators are a deeply committed group of scholarly pioneers who deserve our deepest appreciation for their tilling of new ground for us.

Malcolm S. Knowles, Ph.D.
Professor Emeritus
North Carolina State University

Preface

Each year, physicians, medical colleges, pharmaceutical companies, specialty societies, and hospitals, among many others, spend millions of dollars in pursuit of change. The types of change they seek reflect their unique goals and, occasionally, their special interests. The efficiency of their programs is generally erratic, a function of the variety of assumptions underlying their different approaches to fostering change. Their efforts at change are often based on formalized principles of education, marketing, management, or political science, rather than on knowledge of how resources are integrated and utilized by physicians as they change.

One special interest group, concerned with facilitating change in medicine, saw the value of a clearer and more comprehensive understanding of change as it is perceived by physicians. The Society of Medical College Directors of Continuing Medical Education (SMCDCME) commissioned a wide-ranging study to identify the kinds of changes occurring in physicians' lives, and why and how these changes occurred. The SMCDCME committed its financial resources, as well as the time and effort of many of its members, to developing and conducting this study. It was a collaborative effort, involving a small core of principal investigators, members of the SMCDCME Research Committee, and interviewers and writers from the general membership of the society.

At a meeting of the SMCDCME Research Committee in 1982, the project was initiated by agreement on three research questions involving change in the lives and practices of physicians: (1) What changes have been made, or have occurred? (2) What caused or led up to these changes? (3) Did learning play a role in bringing about these changes? Each member of the Research Committee volunteered to identify two physicians in his or her local area, and to spend approximately one hour with each, asking the research questions, recording responses, and documenting other questions that arose naturally or logically from the interviews. The purpose of the initial interviews was to enable development of an interview guide that could be widely used and would elicit detailed descriptions of the change process. At the next meeting of the research committee, results of these interviews were reported. The research committee's analysis of results was used to continue development of the interview guide, which was further tested by two members of the research committee who assumed leadership for the project. Both members agreed to pilot test the interview guide more extensively in their local areas. In total, forty-four interviews were conducted to test the interview guide. Results of the pilot test were reported to the research committee, and a formal proposal was made for the society to conduct the study.

SMCDCME members sought support for the project from a variety of sources. Primary support for the project was contributed by Med Fund, a foundation of Christ Hospital in Oak Lawn, Illinois. The Upjohn Company was a major contributor. Other contributors included the American College of Cardiology, the American College of Chest Physicians, the American Society of Anesthesiology, the American Society of Clinical Pharmacology and Therapeutics, Clark–O'Neill Mailers, Inc., the Florida Medical Association, the Pennsylvania Medical Society, and the Royal College of Physicians and Surgeons of Canada.

Volunteers from the SMCDCME were asked to conduct interviews within a twenty-mile radius of their medical schools in the United States and Canada. To the extent possible, volunteer interviewers were selected to include disparate and representative geographic regions of North America. Each of the interviewers agreed to participate in training sessions and to conduct and report fifteen interviews within his or her region.

Interviewers were broadly educated about the goals and purpose of the study, and specifically trained in the methods and techniques of the interview. The interview guide provided the fundamental resource questions, but allowed for interaction and probing for details during each interview with physicians.

Acknowledgments

For a project of this size to be successful, more people than could be named must have dedicated their time, energy, and money. The authors received enduring enthusiasm and support from the Society of Medical College Directors of Continuing Medical Education. We are deeply grateful to our colleagues for their understanding, patience, and sponsorship of the Change Study.

Our families have contributed empathy as well as many lost weekends. Our schools have contributed support and encouragement. We are indebted to our staffs for their best efforts, especially Maryann Fuchs and Janice Treadway at East Tennessee State University; Evelyn Hebberd and Kathy Martin at the Medical College of Virginia; and Catherine Nickerson and Kathryn Amero at Dalhousie University.

Our appreciation is extended to George Race, M.D., for challenging us to design the project and to Harold Paul, M.D., for guiding us through its early development. Harold's belief in the importance of this study, and in the abilities of SMCDCME members, helped to inspire Med Fund, a foundation of Christ Hospital in Oak Lawn, Illinois, to provide the bulk of financial support necessary to complete the project.

For our friends at the Upjohn Company and other organizations who also funded a portion of this project, we are very grateful. Those organizations included: American Association of Anesthesiology; American College of Cardiology; American College of Chest Physicians; American Society of Clinical Pharmacology and Therapeutics; Clark-O'Neill Mailers, Inc.; The Educational & Scientific Trust of the Pennsylvania Medical Society; Florida Medical Association; and the Royal College of Physicians & Surgeons of Canada.

Introduction

It may be far simpler to understand *what* doctors change in their professional and personal lives than to understand why and how they do it. This portrait of change in the lives of physicians and the study which forms its foundation were designed to illustrate the how and why. For our purposes, and with apologies to Mr. Webster, a change was viewed as a difference from what was—an alteration in feeling, thought, or action. A definition, however, is only a shadow of the richness and complexity of change, as practicing physicians experience it. What is needed and what we have supplied in this volume is a look at the qualities of changing as they were perceived and reported by the physicians who experienced them. To the best of our knowledge, such a qualitative exploration of change and learning in the lives of physicians never before has been accomplished.

Physicians are good subjects for the study of change. Their attitudes, practices, and lifestyles are products of long, intense education and socialization, which continue even after their formal training ends. The technical nature of their work means that the very basis of their practice, their knowledge, and skills, are constantly changing as their science expands. An ample income presents physicians with diverse opportunities to choose a wide variety of lifestyles and personal situations. Their identity as physicians is pervasive. All of this means that their lives are dynamic and complicated ones, in which changes may be imposed or elected. The changes they experience may be technical or aesthetic, social or personal, complex or simple, and routine or extraordinary.

The types of change doctors make, and the way they make them, are of interest to many different people other than physicians. Patients are interested in the changes that doctors make, because those changes may affect the course of their illness or the costs of their care. Healthcare delivery systems such as hospitals, Health Maintenance Organizations (HMO's), Preferred Provider Organizations (PPO's), and clinics are interested in the changes that physicians make, since these changes directly affect their costs and quality of services. Medical schools and specialty societies have a stake in change in the lives of physicians, because they help create and disseminate the advances of biomedical and behavioral sciences designed to assure progress. Legislators and public officials are also interested in these changes, since their functions are to protect the public from detrimental practices, whether they be ill-advised new procedures or less-than-ideal old procedures. Yet, little is known about how doctors make changes and why. In the absence of knowledge, there are assumptions. It is hoped that by systematically studying change through interviews with a large and diverse sample of physicians, all of the interested stakeholders will have a deeper and more accurate understanding of what, how, and why physicians change.

ABOUT THE STUDY

The idea for this study grew from controversy. At the time of its inception, the single most valued question in continuing medical education (CME) was: "Does CME lead to change?" To answer the question, investigators applied the most time-honored and traditional tools of program planning and research design: The classical program planning model, including needs assessment, objective setting and evaluation, and experimental or quasi-experimental research methods. The strategy was to develop a single educational intervention according to sound principles of program planning, and to verify with proven research tools the effects of the intervention on physician behavior. Results varied and thus, too, conclusions. Sibley et al. (1982) concluded that CME makes no difference. Stein (1981) concluded that it does under certain conditions. Lloyd and Abrahamson (1979) said sometimes it does and sometimes it does not.

What emerged from the myriad studies measuring the impact of CME was an understanding that many variables affecting change in physician behavior were unaccounted-for and difficult to control. It was agreed that rather than looking toward education as a cause, and change as an effect, an alternative approach was necessary. Research efforts should focus on how and why different changes occurred. This would enable an identification of relationships that could explain change in terms of its causes, and describe the role of learning in the change process. The study was to discover a theory of change and learning from systematically collected and analyzed stories of change.

Kerlinger (1973) stated, "Theory is a set of interrelated constructs, definitions and propositions that present a systematic view of phenomena by specifying relations among variables, with the purpose of explaining and predicting phenomena." Experimental, quasi-experimental, correlational, and survey methodologies emphasize verification and testing of specific hypotheses. Only qualitative research methodologies were developed for finding the concrete and conceptual nature of a phenomena. Qualitative research is limited, in that tests of concepts are left for subsequent research. About all that was certain about the nature of change in physicians' lives was that there were questions. We needed to know more about: (1) What changed? (2) Why had it changed? and (3) How did it change?

The first question was qualified with the phrase, "in your life or your practice," to prevent the elimination of information about personal experience. To limit the timespan under consideration, "during the last year" was stipulated, although a few physicians insisted on going as far back as nine years to discuss a change that they felt was currently important in their lives and practices. In its complete form, the first question was, "What changes have you made or have occurred in your life or practice during the past year?"

After each physician described fully *what* had changed, we asked, "What caused this change to occur?" Almost always, physicians offered an explanation in terms of the forces that brought about the change. Some did not, leaning on their scientific background of cautiousness about what *really* causes anything. In some cases, several forces were described as impetuses for change, and in others, only one was viewed as driving the process. In all cases, the descriptions were from the perspectives of those who made the changes or who experienced them. The third fundamental question became, "Did you learn anything in order to make this change?" The question specifically asked for information about how the change process occurred. All the questions reflected certain assumptions about the nature of change. The answers provided valuable insights for those who have a stake in changes in medicine. Understanding how learning is related to changing leads to better ways of designing education to facilitate change. The first question assumed that change is frequent and pervasive for physicians. The second question assumed that something caused these changes. The third question assumed that learning might be instrumental to changing. Although this was not always true, it usually was.

It would be erroneous to assume that circumstances alone control change. With surprising frequency, people change their lives intentionally, and often in areas that are significant—occupation, personal relationships, leisure pursuits, or location of residence. Using an international sample of 150 adults, Tough (1982) indicates only four percent reported making no intentional change during a two-year study period. Changes were often major ones, and the people who made them sought help by reading, consulting with professionals, or talking with other people seen to be helpful. One-third of these changes were related to occupation or profession. The frequency of change reported by Tough has been confirmed in a study of physicians, who are reported to be "constantly involved in making changes in their practice behaviors" (Geertsma 1982, 757).

For most doctors, change is virtually a routine part of life. They do not conceive of professional growth, survival, or competence as apart from seeking or adjusting to change. Physicians see change as a prerequisite for competent medical performance, as a means to achieve life and career goals, and, occasionally, as a response to the unwelcome pressures of modern times. The alternative to controlling the process of change is to be controlled by it, and in dramatic cases, to experience professional or personal collapse.

We knew, if we hoped to understand changes and the process of changing from the viewpoint of physicians, our assumptions would need to be evaluated via a pilot study. Initially, we asked the three questions of five physicians, to probe for additional information and to see if the questions could be answered. The kinds of answers they provided, and their critiques of the questions, allowed us to develop an interview guide for further testing. In the last stage of the pilot study, each member of the SMCDCME Research Committee agreed to conduct two interviews using the interview guide, and to discuss their results with the coinvestigators. The procedures for the study reported in this volume, and the form of interviews, were established as a result of pilot interviews with a total of forty-four physicians. Our intention was to provide a benchmark for future investigations that were accurate, broad-based, and provocative. Thus, we needed to control the quality of the investigations and assure that the results were accurate.

It was agreed that guided interviews with as many physicians as practical, conducted by interviewers from a variety of disciplines (including medicine, behaviorial science, and social science), would best serve exploration of the fundamental research questions and development of research design. All data collection and analysis was oriented toward creating plausible explanations and predictions about the process of change, based in the reality of change in the lives and practices of physicians.

In the spring of 1984, thirteen interviewers from the eastern United States and Canada were trained by the coinvestigators at a session hosted in Boston by Harvard Medical School. Less than a year later, thirteen interviewers from the western United States and Canada were similarly trained at a session hosted by the University of Southern California. Twelve hours of training in the use of the interview guide was accomplished over two days. Interviewers were instructed to begin collecting data within one month after the end of the training session, and were provided with lists representing a random sample of practicing physicians in their geographic areas.

To facilitate the identification of fifteen physicians to be interviewed, a list of seventy-five randomly sampled and sequenced physicians, whose practices were within a twenty-mile radius of the volunteer interviewer's medical school, was provided to each. Each interviewer proceeded down his or her list in order, attempting to contact physicians and arrange interviews. Each interviewer was instructed to make a maximum of three attempts via telephone to contact each respondent to establish an interview time. Interviews were conducted in the offices or work settings of the physicians in nearly all cases. Interviews were scheduled to last one hour, and interviewers were instructed to go completely through the interview guide for each change, repeating the process for subsequent changes, until the hour ended or the physician could no longer recall additional changes. In the 356 interviews conducted, the average number of changes discovered per interview was 2.2. A total of seventy physicians refused to be interviewed. Of all physicians asked to participate in the interviews, 83.5 percent agreed.

Interviewers recorded the results as nearly verbatim as possible. They reported their results in the form of narrative descriptions to provide a look at the whole process of change rather than at specific elements. Quality control of the interviews was accomplished through review of each case narrative by the project director, and by at least one other principal investigator. Cases were discarded for the following conditions:

1. The narrative was internally inconsistent.
2. The interviewer, who had been asked to complete a self-evaluation sheet for each interview, stated that he or she doubted the quality of the interview, or had serious problems with the interviewing situation.
3. Significant data called for in the interview guide were missing from the case.

After cases which failed to meet standards for quality control were eliminated, 775 changes from 340 physicians remained to be analyzed.

The coinvestigators summarized interviewers' narratives, reducing the reports to 4×6 index cards, one for each case of change. These cards formed the basis for conceptualizing forces that produce change, types of changes, and dimensions of learning. Major concepts were confirmed through review of the written narratives. Cards were exchanged among the three coinvestigators to confirm the assignment of each case to the appropriate categories. Assignments to categories were based on similarities and differences between cases. In this way, a broad framework for understanding the 775 changes was developed. In cases where coinvestigators could not agree, the case was discarded. Agreement by the three coinvestigators as to the appropriate category of each case was the final criterion for quality control of information. The process of validation and conceptualization was accomplished in two- to four-day meetings of principal investigators, held four times during the two years of data collection. These meetings were augmented by telephone discussions regarding individual cases.

Because the study was designed to explore and describe change, the focus of analysis was on understanding what physicians *believed* about changes in their lives or their practices. Concepts and categories were based on the recurrence of patterns of interaction among elements of the process of change.

ABOUT THE VOLUME

The remainder of this volume is organized to provide general and specific information about how physicians made changes. Chapter One provides an overview of findings related to major ideas offered in the literature of change and learning in adulthood. Its purpose is to provide an idea framework within which the study can be placed. Chapters Two through Eleven provide detailed views of the changes physicians made according to the forces which drove the processes. Excerpts from the stories of change are used to substantiate how learning relates to specific causes and effects of changing. Each of these chapters begins with a case representing the types of cases of change found within the chapter (informed consent procedures prohibited using verbatim cases, so cases were amalgamated). These chapters close with conclusions and discussions related to changes discussed. Chapter Twelve presents a model and theory of how and why different types of changes occur, as well as a discussion of the potential strengths and weaknesses of this theory. Procedures for developing theory from qualitative data insist that the process be inductive. Placing the theory at the end allows the reader to follow chronologically the movement from specific cases as presented in Chapters Two through Eleven, to general explanations as presented in Chapter Twelve.

This careful process of information collection description was designed not only to identify the attributes and dynamics of change, but also to develop a formal theory which could explain how change and learning are related under different conditions. This theory of change was not only viewed as an important contribution to understanding, but also as a guide for researchers who may seek clearer and more empirically based hypotheses for future research.

REFERENCES

Geertsma, R. H., et al. 1982. How physicians view the process of change in their practice behavior. *Journal of Medical Education* 57:752–768.

Kerlinger, F. 1973. *Foundations of behavioral research*. New York: Holt, Rinehart, and Winston.

Lloyd, J. S., and S. Abrahamson. 1979. The effectivenesss of continuing medical education: A review of the evidence. *Evaluation in the Health Professions* 2:251–280.

Sibley, J. C., et al. 1982. A randomized trial of continuing medical education. *The New England Journal of Medicine* 306:511–515.

Stein, L. S. 1981. The effectiveness of continuing medical education: Eight research reports. *Journal of Medical Education* 56:103–110.

Tough, A. 1982. *Intentional Changes: A fresh approach to helping people change*. Chicago: Follett Publ. Co.

1

An Overview

Robert D. Fox,
Paul E. Mazmanian,
and R. Wayne Putnam

A body of theory about the ways that people make changes in their lives must rest on a base of careful explorations. There have been only a few field studies of people as they learn and change, and these investigations have not been designed to support a comprehensive theory of the phenomena that have been studied. Too often this kind of research has reported findings that are really untested assumptions or theoretical constructs, rather than data. Consequently, there is little in the way of natural history to guide our thinking about a ubiquitous process in adult life.

In this study of change and learning in physicians' lives, we have committed ourselves to developing, first, a descriptive natural history of our subject, and second, a taxonomy of our observations. No such undertaking begins in a vacuum, of course. Ideas and theories of how adults alter themselves and their behaviors do exist. And, in any case, a major effort is made to teach and change physicians throughout their lives through continuing medical education (CME) (Cervero 1988). The practice of CME is both tacitly and explicitly based on notions about the way learning modifies behavior.

From the transcripts of our interviews with physicians, we were able to identify three elements for integration into an explanatory model:

1. People do not alter themselves or their lives arbitrarily—they have reasons. We have sought to classify these reasons, which we characterize as *forces* tending to bring about change.

2. Changes are not automatically achieved. The adult who alters his or her way of doing business with the world must usually acquire new knowledge and skills. We have analyzed the types and forms of *learning* that helped our subjects to make their changes.

3. Changes may range from the minor (grudging acquiescence) to the all-encompassing (changes of career, lifestyles, and relationships). In part, but only in part, this element of change can be characterized as a matter of magnitude—measured, perhaps, in the number of minutes or hours in the day that are affected by it. But it is more realistic to recognize that quality and magnitude are combined in the subjective experience of conditions "now" versus "then"—and in resistance to it or willingness to embrace it. When we speak of *types* of change, it is this difference that we have in mind: The extent to which actions overcome inertia and obstacles to result in altered behavior and consciousness.

In the remainder of this chapter, we will review our observations in light of some popular and theoretical notions about change and learning.

FORCES FOR CHANGE

A convenient summary of the major analyses of behavior change distinguishes between the *mechanistic* and the *organismic* approaches (Green 1984). The main proponents of the mechanistic approach are behaviorists, who stress the role of environmental reinforcement and punishment as the determinants of change. The individual, in this model, works in a fairly mechanical way to minimize discomfort and maximize rewards. Forces are external, responses are internal. The organismic alternative, for example, in cognitive theory, finds forces within the person as well. Values or preferences become attached to an anticipated future— the tension, between things as they are and things as they might become, is a force driving the person to change. Green (1984), in summarizing, uses the terms "intrinsic" and "extrinsic" motivation: "Intrinsic motivation comes from within the individual and is comprised of urges, wishes, feelings, emotions, desires, and drives. Extrinsic motivation comes from outside the individual and is manifest in those environmental factors that precipitate behavior."

These approaches are not, of course, mutually exclusive. Both incorporate a notion of conflict as the underlying inducement to make a change. Lewin (1951) has generalized more broadly about the ways that a resolution of forces may either maintain stability or precipitate behavior leading to change. The distinction between internal and external is less important in his formulation—factors in the social environment may conflict or conspire in ways that force a change, and so may tendencies within the individual. The sense of imbalance and anxiety, produced by the pressure and counterpressure of such forces, serves as the driving motivation for change.

A recent review of continuing education in the professions (Nowlen 1988) suggests that the performance of physicians is structured by a double helix, in which there are two complex interactive strands—one carrying cultural influences, the other carrying the individuals' characteristics. The culture-based strand carries the history, values, mission, character, style, symbols, resources, and structures of each culture in which an individual moves. It carries each culture's performance expectations, motivation, recognition, reward, and punishment. The strand representing individual-based performance carries information from the individuals' lifetimes of prior cultural interactions, from every context within which meaning was developed and growth took place. It carries the individual's attributes, limitations and predispositions. The pairing of the strands, matched or mismatched, results in performance.

Often our subjects did not distinguish clearly between personal and environmental factors that induced them to change. Rather, they identified most of their changes as a response to professional concerns, more or less lumping extrinsic and intrinsic motives. This finding doesn't really invalidate the distinction, however. Becoming a physician entails a long and intensive process of socialization, one that begins well before medical school (Harville 1981). What a doctor is, or must be, is established in society by law and regulation, within the profession by formal codes as well as informally by the attitudes of teachers and colleagues, by patients' expectations, and through popular characterizations in journalism and fiction. When medical education succeeds, the externally defined role becomes an accepted component of self-definition, owned by the student or graduate physician, but occupying a territory that is at the intersection of personal values and social imperatives.

Professionalism, the internalized set of socially generated expectations, becomes itself a permanent, discrete, and powerful agent for change. Physicians in our sample identified purely professional motivations as driving the largest fraction of changes they made. These were the desire for enhanced competence (24 percent) and the perception that their clinical environment pressed for a change (14 percent). Other reasons for change shaded away from this professional core toward more social or personal motivations. Personal desires could be mixed with professional goals, as in an effort to improve financial status (9 percent), or to move on to a further stage of career development (8 percent). Somewhat less often, purely personal considerations were cited, for example, their personal well-being (8 percent) or pure curiosity (4 percent). Likewise, professional motives could become increasingly mixed with social pressures: Relationships with colleagues in the same institution (11 percent), or the profession (9 percent), or a felt need to respond to regulations (10 percent). Roles in the family or the community, outside any professional context, accounted for only five percent of all the changes we heard described.

Not all forces impel change, of course. Some deter it. Many of our subjects cited factors inhibiting change. Regardless of the arena in which the pressure for change was felt, strong counterforces might be described, and these sometimes caused intense conflict. Our interviews were not structured specifically to elicit descriptions of opposition to change; if they had been, its importance might have been more pronounced in our results.

Whether change was easy or difficult often depended on the context in which it was made, and the physician's perception of the reasons for changing. As Bennis, Benne, and Chin (1985) have observed, behavior is rather easily modified when the result is perceived as rational, relatively easy to achieve, and in the best interest of the person. The physicians in our sample identified many small, fairly simple changes that they made to improve their clinical competence, and they expressed satisfaction with these changes. But when change is coerced rather than induced (or perceived as such), opposition and dissatisfaction are probable results. Although the threat of punishment can propel change, for example, attempts at regulation, the response is likely to be minimal and grudging.

Larger and more complex changes, on the other hand, are more often associated with a positive emotional tone. Such changes are often associated with personal motivations—to satisfy curiosity, to enhance well-being, or to advance one's career or social position. In general, the pattern we observed supports the theory of affective arousal, that "affect is the basis of motivation in that it precedes, energizes and directs behavior" (McClelland 1953; in Green 1984, 58).

Even when the forces for change are in place, and favor it, a triggering event may be required (Geertsma 1982). A personal crisis, such as illness or depression, might serve the purpose in the personal sphere. A professional response might be facilitated by the introduction of an innovation in technology, or by a particular patient's problem. Socially motivated change often was triggered by the opening of a career opportunity or a request for help from one's colleagues or institution. Whatever its source, a triggering event appears to attenuate the difficulty of initiating change.

What our study may add to the existing body of ideas about the forces of change is that the distinction between intrinsic and extrinsic forces is insufficient. Professionalism, with its peculiar fusion of personal identity and social role, may act as a third, and somewhat self-propelling reason for change. The physicians in our sample changed for reasons that fall on a spectrum from the highly personal, to the professional, to the purely social. The changes were more vigorous, complex, and happy when they were perceived as arising from within rather than as being coerced. And a triggering event was often identifiable.

LEARNING AS A RESPONSE

Behavior change may be achieved without a sustained period of overt learning, however; in the stories physicians told us, learning was generally central to the process. In just under thirty percent of cases, physicians claimed to have done no learning, but simply to have made a change for which they already possessed the knowledge and skill. This response was particularly evident when the force for change was mainly social.

It is hardly surprising that over two-thirds of the changes we recorded involved some kind of learning, although the reason that learning is so central may not be as obvious as it seems. Theories about why adults learn are more developed than theories of how they learn, but consensus has not been achieved (Merriam 1987). Learning often is seen as a native feature of adulthood (andragogy), but there are also complex models hinging on the psychology of motivation (for example, path-goal theory).

The concept of andragogy (one of the most influential and widespread accounts of the who and how of adult learning) is based on four truisms:

1. maturation is a natural transition from dependence to independence,

2. increased experience becomes a natural resource for further learning in adulthood,

3. development of new social roles imposes a need to learn, and

4. learning can be applied in increasingly immediate and important ways to adult problems (Knowles 1980).

The validity of these truisms has been tested by Tough (1978, 1982), who has explored the learning projects undertaken by adults, and intentional changes made in adult lives. He investigated the deliberate efforts of adults "to gain and retain certain definite knowledge and skills or to change in some other way". He found that one-third were related to occupation, and that learning was integral to the process. Both Knowles and Tough have observed that adults do learn in ways they plan and direct for themselves, but an explicit theory of change has not emerged from their works.

The physicians in our study fit rather well with earlier observations. They learned independently in response to goals they set themselves, and they embedded learning in the process of change. The imperative to learn appeared to be part of their identification with their social role.

Most provocative from earlier studies of adult learning is the emphasis on problem solving (Knowles 1975). Our subjects commonly did use learning to solve concrete problems, but they also very often sought to gain broader understanding of a subject. At both extremes of motivation to change, when responding to personal curiosity or when coping with the new structure of regulations, they were quite likely to seek a conceptual grasp of the subject. Granted, a "problem" might be seen at the heart of the effort to learn and change, but in about forty-one percent of our cases, understanding seemed to be given a higher priority than the immediate solution to the problem.

A more longitudinal characterization of learning has been developed by Cross (1981), who identifies a sequence of elements affecting the decision to initiate one episode of learning, the act of learning itself, and consequences for future episodes. The model begins with a person who has a certain self-evaluation, and a set of attitudes about education, which then combine with an estimate of the importance of certain goals and expectations of success, through learning. The salience of the goals is affected by transitions in life; opportunities to learn and barriers to doing so interact with these other factors, depending, in part, on how much information is available about them. The status of these factors affects participation in learning. Eventually, the outcome of that learning loops back to influence the person's self-evaluation and attitudes toward education. This model draws heavily on the path-goal model of motivation (Vroom 1964). This is a model of the way that adults assess the value of achieving their goals (valence), and their level of expectancy (the estimated probability of achieving the goal), as a way of deciding how much of their resources to expend in an effort to achieve those goals. Like any theory of motivation, of course, the model infers what must be in the "black box" controlling human behavior, as the process itself is not accessible to direct observation (Green 1984).

We find some correspondences between the accounts our physicians gave us and Cross's model, at least, in the ways that the components of motivation to change were identified. In their narratives, the doctors linked their changes to episodes of self-evaluation and the effects of transitions in their lives. Their accounts, of both opportunities for, and barriers to change, are ubiquitous. Their patterns of learning were adjusted to the anticipated change—the amount was greater when the change was perceived as coming from within, less when it was seen as coerced. We obtained relatively little information about the doctors' attitudes toward education because they volunteered little, and the reality appeared to be that most of their learning efforts went on outside formal programs. Because the primary focus of this study was on change rather than learning, we have a relatively rich view of the way learning was integrated into the process of change, but not much information about learning for reasons other than change.

Another facet of the motivation to learn is the focus of Knox's proficiency theory (Merriam 1987). This exceedingly rational view of motivation holds that a person assesses the level of proficiency required for a given situation, compares it to the existing level, and then takes measures to reduce the disparity. This very straightforward model is at the heart of many applied programs in CME, to the extent that such programs are based on "assessment of need" (Fox 1983). Proficiency theory, simple as it is, is not free of theoretical problems. For example, how large a gap between present and desirable proficiency is needed to stimulate learning? Fiske and Maddi (in Knox 1977) have suggested that some discrepancies are too small to provoke action. Very large gaps, on the other hand, may create too much anxiety, leading to denial, avoidance, or a shift in one's estimate of what ought to be (Knox 1977).

Again, because proficiency theory offers an account of what goes on inside a person's head, it is not verifiable from direct observation. Indirectly, however, our findings offer some support for it, primarily when our subjects expressed the wish to become more competent. Repeatedly, we heard them talk about wanting to be better doctors, or more "up to date." On the other hand, they also appeared to learn and make changes in areas where they already felt competent, although this was often in response to external demands—regulations, income, family responsibilities—and the demands of patients. On balance, there was far more direct support for the notion that learning is driven by some kind of internal comparison of present and projected states than for other motivations. Of course, one way to circumvent the "black box" problem is to ask people directly why they do something. The accuracy of the answers depends on the respondents' ability to describe their motivations accurately, but it shouldn't be assumed a priori that this is impossible. Indeed, a theoretical premise of our study is that learners can interpret and articulate their reasons for learning. "If men define situations as real, they are real in their consequences" (Thomas 1970, 154). This sociological axiom underlies our approach—people's perception of reality is what governs their behavior, not necessarily an "objective" reality.

With respect to learning, the direct approach most often has been used in assessing reasons for participating in formal education programs. Houle (1961) initiated this kind of research by asking active learners their reasons for taking courses. Richards' review (1980) of this topic identified six reasons that doctors give for learning:

1. it is part of being a professional,
2. the subject matter is interesting,
3. they are validating previous experience,
4. they are attaining specific objectives,
5. they need a change of pace, or
6. they want more social contact.

We can't add much to this list because our study focused only on learning as part of the process of changing, but our findings certainly support the first three items (professionalism, curiosity, and desire for competence) as reasons for learning.

LEARNING AS A PROCESS

Most ideas about how adults learn fall short of being specific and complete theories. Mostly, they are presented as a collection of theory-like statements (a notable exception is Kolb's (1976) experiential theory of learning). Some salient questions about learning in adult life remain to be answered. How, if at all, do adults differ from children in their approaches to learning? Do people differ in their style of learning, and are the differences a relatively stable feature of personality? More attention has been directed to comparing the *ability* of adults and children to learn than to analyzing their respective methods of learning. Knowles (1978), in looking at the differences between the way adults and children approach learning, has contended that the greater experience and independence of adults leads them to be more "self-directed" than children.

Manning and DeBakey (1988) interviewed selected physicians to develop descriptions of their personal and moral traits, as well as the ways they stay abreast of advances in modern medicine. The authors provided valuable information on the lives of medical leaders, and on the personal and professional rewards of lifelong learning. They describe reading and consulting, to obtain information used to solve questions arising in practice, as learning methods. To these fundamental strategies, they add discussions with peers and mentors, practice audits, teaching, writing, and reassessing information as useful ways to learn. With their work, Manning and DeBakey confirm that recent advances in computer technology can facilitate and expand the benefits of traditional approaches to learning. Their study offers helpful insight into the learning activities of doctors, but it does not, and was not intended, to offer a set of statements that can help predict how physicians learn and change under specific conditions.

Houle (1980) offers a typology for describing professionals' continuous learning activities. He identifies three "major and overlapping modes of learning," labeled inquiry, instruction, and performance. In inquiry, " . . . learning is a by-product (though sometimes an intended by-product) of efforts directed primarily at establishing policy, seeking consensus, working out compromises, and projecting plans." He defines instruction as "the process of disseminating established skills, knowledge, or sensitiveness." Performance is defined as "the process of internalizing an idea or using a practice habitually, so that it becomes a fundamental part of the way in which a learner thinks about and undertakes his or her work." Cervero and Dimmock (1987) tested the extent to which Houle's framework is an accurate description of the structural forms of professionals' continuing learning activities. They surmise that his mode of instruction may be differentiated into group instruction and self-instruction. The stories physicians told us certainly supported the notion that they learn autonomously, but the quality of "self-directedness" eludes measurement. We found nothing to contradict the notion that adults' learning is self-directed, but, of course, we were not comparing adults with children, just as we were not comparing people of different classes or professions.

We might, however, have expected to see some differences in learning style as defined by experiential learning theory. As developed by Kolb (1976), this model offers a systematic view of differences in people's preferred strategies of learning. Two orthogonal dimensions are the framework of the theory. Along one axis, people range in their preference for abstract, categorical notions of the world, versus concrete, specific descriptions. Along the other axis, learners distribute themselves according to their preferred role. Reflective observers are at one extreme; active participants are at the other. The two perpendicular axes define four quadrants, which can be characterized as *learning* styles, *relatively stable* preferences for a particular approach to learning. These preferences are, in turn, driven by attributes of personality, such as cognitive style (Kolb 1976). Efforts to validate the questionnaire developed by Kolb to elicit learning styles have challenged the instrument (Fox 1983), but many scholars in the field continue to accept these two dimensions as capturing some quality of reality. Yet it remains unclear whether adults consistently exhibit one or another learning style. As we analyzed our own findings, we found that the way physicians characterized their involvement in learning lent itself to a typology with three dimensions: the *purpose* for which learning was undertaken, the *method* of learning, and the *resources* that were used.

Although all instances of learning that we recorded were initiated for the purpose of making a change in life or in medical practice, the intention in some cases was to develop and integrate concepts that would raise one's general level of understanding, whereas in other cases, the intention was to solve a specific problem. In nearly two-thirds of the instances we recorded, learning was intended to solve a particular problem, as opposed to the more general aim of enhancing understanding.

Somewhat analogously to Kolb's distinction between reflective and active approaches to learning, we were able to distinguish between physicians who preferred hands-on, participatory learning and those who organized their activities to facilitate a more reflective approach. We distinguished these as "experiential" and "deliberative" methods of learning. In real life, of course, such methods could not be purely applied, but it was generally possible to classify a physician's approach to learning as predominantly either experiential (for example, observing and practicing a new surgical technique) or deliberative (for example, evaluating the literature on intensive home monitoring of blood sugar in diabetes). In the instances we recorded, each strategy predominated about half the time.

Schon's (1987) concept of reflection in action presents an alternative look at learning methods, considering them a conceptual component of a continuous reflective conversation with the practice situation, including problem setting, the process by which the professional defines the decision to be made, the ends to be achieved, and the means which may be chosen. The reflective act of practice is the elemental structure of self-directed learning in the professions. It is so much a piece of each professional act that it is virtually impossible to distinguish action from reflection. Each reflective act is a teaching-learning situation. Schon's approach includes an inner voice that occupies a higher level of conscious learning, higher than the fundamentally structured reflections. The inner voice "marks" certain ideas, exchanges, events, strategies, tactics, and examples for subsequent reflection, acting in concert with the practitioner's other voice, which interacts directly with the situation at play (Schon 1987).

Deliberate but simple acts, such as subscribing to journals or registering for the annual meeting of a specialty society comprise the next highest level of conscious involvement. At the highest level of intentionality are complex learning projects undertaken with personal and organizational outcomes in view, and typically mixing self-managed learning experiences with provider-directed programs in an overarching framework that is, itself, largely self-designed (Schon 1983). The number and variety of resources that physicians use for learning makes classification in this dimension more difficult. The task was complicated by the fact that doctors have their own tacit ways of classifying resources, for example, by distinguishing between the "good" journal and the "throwaway," or by discriminating between consultants, some of whom are defined as "experts." The underlying polarity that we found, however, was between resources that received explicit endorsement from professional or academic bodies, versus those that were seen as useful, but lacked any kind of sanction (such as CME credit). Overall, learning relied on formal resources in about two-thirds of the cases we recorded.

We could ask of these data whether patterns of learning were influenced more by personality or more by the situation that elicited the activity, because 130 of our subjects described between two and six instances of learning. The choice of either purpose *or* method was consistent in only one-fifth of these cases, of purpose *and* method only about one time in seven. If learning preferences are chiefly determined by personality, a higher degree of consistency should have emerged. By contrast, a systematic connection was observed between the purpose given for learning and the type of force impelling the learning to take place. The more internal the motivation for learning, the more likely it was to be approached conceptually; external forces brought about the type of learning that was associated with specific problem solving, as Figure 1 shows. Likewise, the method chosen varied with the motivation. Learning was more likely to be experiential when the pressures for change were described as purely professional, more likely to be deliberative when the pressure was purely social, as Figure 2 shows.

Formal rather than informal resources were used on three-quarters of the occasions when the learning was done in response to professional needs. Informal resources were more likely to be used when the cause of change was personal, social, or a mixture of personal and professional, as Figure 3 shows. The following chapters give a more detailed view of the way in which the approaches to learning varied with the force to which the physicians were responding.

EDUCATION AND CHANGE

To this point, our view of learning has been centered in the physician, the person who is doing it (and this has governed our choice of words). Education is, of course, intended to bring about learning, but through an externally designed and, often, imposed structure. However partial, tacit, and informal *theories* of learning may be, they are inevitably converted into a formal structure of *practice* when courses of instruction are designed. Thus, curricula for CME imply by their very design a set of principles about physicians, their motivations for learning, and the means by which it is most effectively accomplished. Prescriptions for CME have been developed in advance of obtaining validated descriptions.

The essential concepts in the current planning of CME are *needs, objectives, programs,* and *impacts,* which form a linear progression in the model of optimal curriculum design.

Needs assessment — Objectives — CME program — Change

When this model is effectively realized, the physician's needs for new knowledge or skill are measured, behavioral objectives are designed to reduce the discrep-

Figure 1.1
Purpose of Learning According to Force for Change

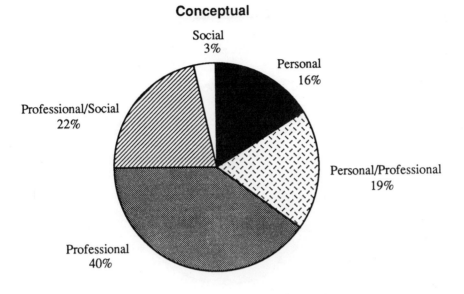

Conceptual

Social 3%

Personal 16%

Professional/Social 22%

Personal/Professional 19%

Professional 40%

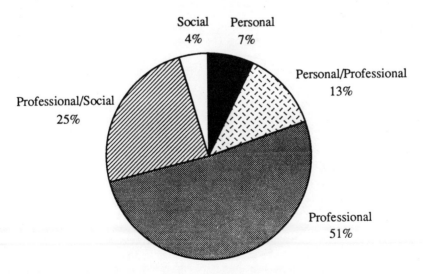

Problem Specific

Social 4% Personal 7%

Personal/Professional 13%

Professional/Social 25%

Professional 51%

Figure 1.2
Learning Method According to Force for Change

Experiential

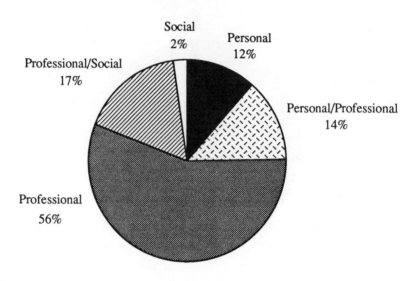

Social 2%

Personal 12%

Professional/Social 17%

Personal/Professional 14%

Professional 56%

Deliberative

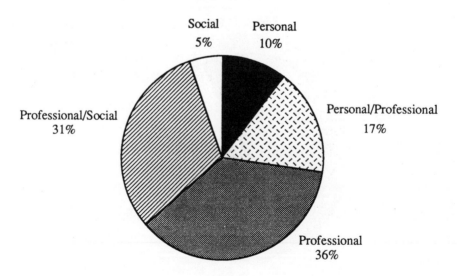

Social 5%

Personal 10%

Professional/Social 31%

Personal/Professional 17%

Professional 36%

Figure 1.3
Learning Resources According to Force for Change

Formal

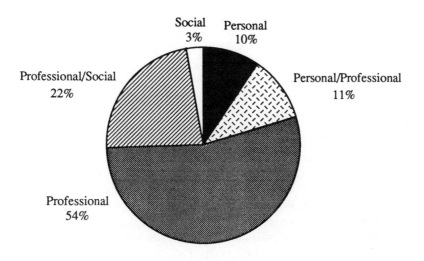

Social 3%

Personal 10%

Professional/Social 22%

Personal/Professional 11%

Professional 54%

Informal

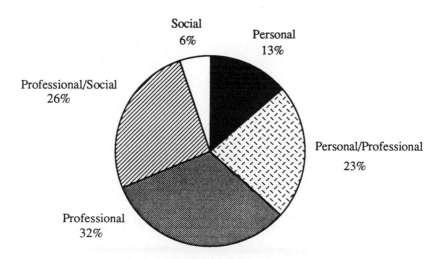

Social 6%

Personal 13%

Professional/Social 26%

Personal/Professional 23%

Professional 32%

ancies, and a controlled learning experience is designed and provided, after which, the enrollees change their behavior and therefore their patients' health status. That this model is accepted virtually without question probably stems from the medical model itself: Diagnosis leads to treatment, which is followed by cure. The accreditation system now in place for CME programs, leaning heavily on this model, requires assessment of needs, preparation of objectives, and evaluation of programs. It stops, however, at the much more difficult task of assessing the effect of changed behavior on patient outcomes, and studies of this all-important aspect of CME have yielded mixed results.

Bertram and Brooks-Bertram (1971) reviewed the literature and concluded that, in most circumstances, the methodology of such evaluations have been flawed, but, even when they were appropriate, yielded mixed results. Lloyd and Abrahamson (1979) reviewed forty-seven studies published since 1962, thirty of them since 1940. Changes in physicians' performance were evaluated in twenty-six of the studies, mostly through chart audit. Of these twenty-six studies, eleven reported positive change, eight reported no change, and seven reported a mix of positive and negative changes. Of the total of forty-seven studies, only two examined both actual performance and competencies, and only four examined health status of patients. The reviewers concluded that there was little evidence to support the claim that CME has a direct effect on physicians' competence or performance, let alone on the health status of their patients. Five years later, Haynes et al. (1984) reviewed 248 original articles evaluating CME. Only seven of these met their methodological standards, and all of these provided convincing evidence that CME can improve the behavior of physicians, but only three of them assessed patient outcomes, and of these, only one showed any improvement.

Two more recent studies, one by Dunn et al. (1988), and one by Wergin et al. (1988), reported somewhat conflicting results. Dunn et al. found there were no relationships between quality of care and either the type or quantity of physicians' CME activities. Wergin et al. indicated that change attributable to CME was generally subtle and often delayed. CME courses had a significant impact on the behavior of practicing physicians, when behavior change was defined to include refinements in patient care, not just wholesale practice changes. They suggested that research in CME needs to focus more explicitly on attitudes, intentions, and the social context of physician practices. The researchers concluded that those responsible for designing and implementing CME must consider alternatives to the current CME model, in order to free themselves from trying to document whether or not an isolated even of CME changes physician practice behavior.

The model of CME may or may not be valid as it applies to the design of educational programs, but it hardly captures the reality of the way doctors make changes in their lives and practices. Education is indeed one of the resources that doctors use, especially when they are focusing on their clinical competence, or are responding to changes in the clinical environment, but it is not necessarily a pivotal resource. Educational experiences are complemented by other sources of information and instruction, both before and after changes are made. When change is driven by highly personal or highly social influences, formal education plays an insignificant role, and learning on the whole is minimal.

TOWARD A TAXONOMY OF LEARNING AND CHANGE

Changes are not all alike. It may well be that progress in understanding the ways people make changes in their lives has been retarded by a failure to distinguish adequately among types of change. We hoped in this investigation to explore some of the differences in the way people change. In our data, one aspect of change that has defied classification consists of the various objects of change. Physicians, for example, might change the way they speak, prescribe, listen, examine, view, or feel; the change might be directed toward patients, clinics, drugs, equipment, relationships, procedures, rules, and so on. The "and so on" was our problem; such a large array was cataloged in this study that we found no effective way to categorize the objects of change.

However, we were able to extract a classification of changes that was based on the nature of the difference between "now" and "then". The four parts of this classification were labeled *accommodation* (126 instances), *adjustment* (481), *redirection* (141), and *transformation* (27). Three criteria were used for deciding which of these categories a change belonged to. These were:

magnitude as defined by how much change was made, *complexity* from incremental to structural, and *attitude,* chiefly positive or negative.

A visual representation of the classification is given below.

TYPES OF CHANGE ACCORDING TO SIZE, COMPLEXITY, AND ATTITUDE

	SIZE	COMPLEXITY	ATTITUDE
Accomodation	Small	Simple	Compliant, often accompanied by negative feelings
Adjustment	Small to moderate	Incremental	Little emotion but usually positive when expressed
Redirection	Large	Structural, major element	Moderate to strong emotion usually positive
Transformation	Large	Complex, Involving many inter-relationships	Very strong emotions usually positive

Accommodation was typically the type of change requiring a small and simple act of acceptance, and such a change often elicited a neutral or negative reaction. Changes of this type were highly focused and seldom went beyond the immediate area to other aspects of behavior or attitude. For example, a physician might be required to adopt a new informed consent procedure by the hospital. Compliance might be rapid and simple, with a neutral or somewhat irritated response.

Adjustment was similarly brought to pass with little emotion, but this type of change required a more complex adaptation and more time and effort to accomplish. To continue with the example of a consent form, adjustment might entail the physician's feeling that the new form was more appropriate, learning about the rationale, and using it to engage in a different, more meaningful level of discussion with patients. Adjustments were characterized by an active assessment of the disparity, or fit, between what is and what ought to be, by considered and purposeful behavior directed to that end.

Redirection required adding, subtracting, or changing a major element of one's life or practice, and usually was accompanied with moderately to strongly positive feelings. For example, a physician might, with relief, decide to abandon the practice of obstetrics but remain in gynecology because of dissatisfaction with the state of malpractice insurance and litigation affecting obstetrics.

Transformation required restructuring and redefinition of many elements in the physician's personal or professional life. For example, a physician might come to enjoy the counseling activities associated with informed consent. Coming to see this as a special skill may lead to a return to residency training in order to switch to a specialty which allows for more of this kind of interaction. All 775 changes that we recorded could be assigned to one of these four categories, with agreement among the three of us. But naturally enough a few cases were more blurry than others.

We apologize for introducing a new set of terms or concepts into a muddled jargon, but we saw no alternative. First, the terms arose from our data—they correspond to what the physicians described in their interviews. Second, we were not able to find an existing set of terms in the literature that corresponded to our observations, with one exception. Mezirow (1981) has looked at a phenomenon that he labels "perspective transformation". Our use of the term differs from his in that we use only the outcome (the difference between the subject's status before and after the change is complete) to decide whether a transformation has occurred. Mezirow's definition includes elements of process as well as outcome. Also unlike Mezirow, we did not evaluate the outcome (for example, as "personal liberation") in deciding whether a change was a transformation or not.

Another second-order distinction between the various types of change had to do with whether learning was required. In many cases, the inducement to change came with a more-or-less automatic prescription for the way in which it was to be accomplished, and no learning was reported. Alternatively, the incentive to change, and ideas about what kind of change was indicated, motivated learning, through which the change was accomplished.

PATTERNS AND CONTEXTS

The various taxonomic characteristics that we have identified as forces, forms of learning, and types of outcome are not randomly associated with one another. Accommodation, for example, was most likely to be a response to social or professional forces (for example, regulations), and required little learning. Learning was required in only about two-fifths of these cases, as compared with almost three-quarters of the total. The type of learning was about equally problem specific or conceptual, and was deliberative rather than experiential in fifty-four percent of cases. These proportions differ little from the trend in our sample as a whole. There was somewhat more resort to informal than formal learning resources (51 percent) with this type of change than in all changes (34 percent).

Adjustment was generally a response to professional forces. Purely professional considerations, the desire to increase competence or respond to the clinical environment, occasioned nearly half the changes in this category. And, correspondingly, the response to a professional pressure for change was most often an adjustment (77 percent of such cases). Three-quarters of these changes entailed some learning, which differed little in its characteristics from the entire sample.

Redirection was more commonly a response to personal forces than either acceptance or adjustment and was less likely to be a response to professional or social forces. Curiosity and desire for personal well-being accounted for a quarter of such changes. Learning took place in over three quarters of redirections and was again typical of the sample as a whole.

Transformations were rare, but one statistic stands out and is probably meaningful: Only one of twenty-seven transformations occurred in response to a purely professional force. Learning was part of twenty-two such cases and tended to be time-consuming, complex, and conceptual in character.

Our study of change and learning in the lives and practices of physicians was not designed as a follow-up or expansion on the works of others, but our findings do connect to some of the major ideas about adult learning and change. In spite of these points of connection, this study also makes several unique contributions. First, the investigation emphasized similarities and differences among forces, learning strategies, and changes. Discovering how these components of the change process differ is instrumental to explaining and predicting changes. We hope the explanations and predictions found in subsequent chapters will help to advance research and educational practices directed towards change. The concepts and propositions we offer are built from the narratives of change provided by our subjects. They were collected expressly for the purpose of building theory grounded in life experiences. We believe that this perspective will facilitate more

Figure 1.4
Accommodation Changes According to Force for Change

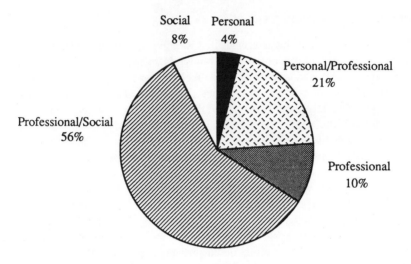

Accomodations

Social
8%

Personal
4%

Personal/Professional
21%

Professional/Social
56%

Professional
10%

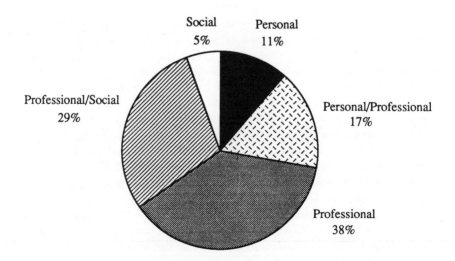

All Changes

Social
5%

Personal
11%

Professional/Social
29%

Personal/Professional
17%

Professional
38%

Figure 1.5
Adjustments According to Force for Change

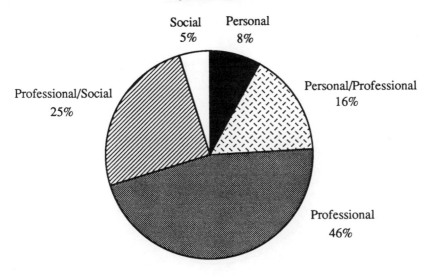

Adjustments

Social
5%

Personal
8%

Personal/Professional
16%

Professional/Social
25%

Professional
46%

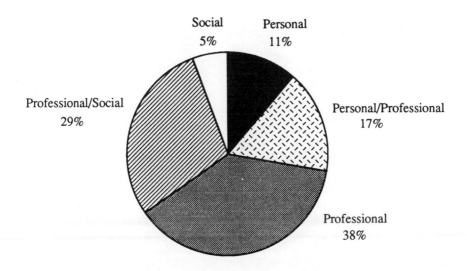

All Changes

Social
5%

Personal
11%

Professional/Social
29%

Personal/Professional
17%

Professional
38%

Figure 1.6
Redirections According to Force for Change

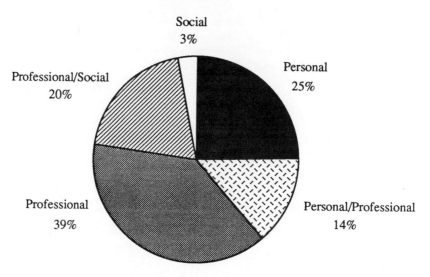

Redirections

Social
3%

Personal
25%

Professional/Social
20%

Professional
39%

Personal/Professional
14%

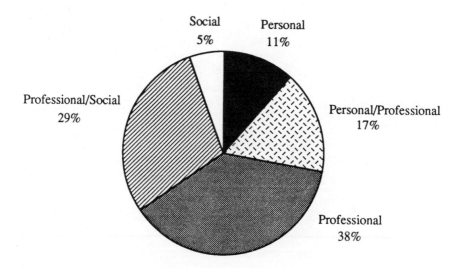

All Changes

Social
5%

Personal
11%

Professional/Social
29%

Personal/Professional
17%

Professional
38%

research and better educational practices without sacrificing the authentic qualities of these stories of change and learning.

The next ten chapters describe changes according to the ten specific forces precipitating change. In each, the authors attempt not only to preserve the en vivo qualities of their cases but also to discover the ideas which contribute to the similarities and differences among them. The final chapter describes a set of theoretical propositions and a model which describes the overall relationship between forces for change, learning, and types of changes.

REFERENCES

Bennis, W., K. Benne, and R. Chin. 1985. *The planning of change*. 4th ed. New York: Holt, Rinehart, and Winston.

Bertram, D. A., and P. A. Brooks-Bertram. 1971. The evaluation of continuing medical education: A literature review. *Health Education Monographs* 5:330–348.

Cervero, R. M. 1988. *Effective continuing education for professionals*. San Francisco: Jossey-Bass Publishers.

Cervero, R. M., and K. H. Dimmock. 1987. A factor analytic test of Houle's typology of professional's models of learning. *Adult Education Quarterly* 37:125–129.

Cross, P. K. 1981. *Adults as learners*. San Francisco: Jossey-Bass Publishers.

Dunn, E. V., et al. 1988. Study of relation of continuing medical education to quality of family physicians' care. *Journal of Medical Education* 63:775–784.

Fox, R. D. 1983. Discrepancy analysis of continuing medical education: A conceptual model. *Mobius* 3:37–44.

Geertsma, R. H., et al. 1982. How physicians view the process of change in their practice behavior. *Journal of Medical Education* 57:752–768.

Green, J. S., et al., eds. 1984. *Continuing education for the health professions: Developing, managing, and evaluating programs for maximum impact on patient care*. San Francisco: Jossey-Bass Publishers.

Harvill, L. M. 1981. Anticipatory socialization of medical students. *Journal of Medical Education* 56:431–433.

Haynes, R. B., et al. 1984. A critical reappraisal of the efficacy of continuing medical education. *Journal of the American Medical Association* 251:61–64.

Houle, C. O. 1961. *The inquiring mind*. Madison: The University of Wisconsin Press.

———. 1980. *Continuing learning in the professions*. San Francisco: Jossey-Bass Publishers.

Knowles, M. S. 1975. *Self-directed learning: A guide for learners and teachers*. Chicago: Association Press.

———. 1978. *The adult learner: A neglected species*. Houston, Texas: Gulf Publ. Co.

———. 1980. *The modern practice of adult education*. Chicago: Follett Press.

Knox, A. B. 1977. *Adult development and learning: A handbook on individual growth and competence in the adult years for education in the helping professions*. San Francisco: Jossey-Bass.

Kolb, D. A. 1976. *Learning style inventory technical manual*. Boston: McBee and Co.

Lewin, K. 1951. *Field theory in social science*. New York: Harper and Row.

Lloyd, J. S., and S. Abrahamson. 1979. The effectiveness of continuing medical education: A review of the evidence. *Evaluation in the Health Professions* 2:251–280.

McClelland, D. C., et al. 1953. *The achievement motive.* New York: Appleton-Century-Crofts. In Green, J. S., et al. 1984. *Continuing education for the health professions.* San Francisco: Jossey-Bass Publishers.

Manning, P. R., and L. DeBakey. 1988. *Medicine: Preserving the passion.* New York: Springer-Verlag.

Merriam, S. B. 1987. Adult learning and theory building: A review. *Adult Education Quarterly* 37:187–198.

Mezirow, J. 1981. A critical theory of adult learning and education. *Adult Education* 32:3–24.

Nowlen, P. M. 1988. *A new approach to continuing education for business and the professions.* New York: Macmillan.

Richards, R. K., and R. M. Cohen. Why physicians attend traditional CME programs. *Journal of Medical Education* 55:479–485.

Schon, D. A. 1983. *The reflective practitioner.* New York: Basic Books.

———. 1987. *Educating the reflective practitioner.* San Francisco: Jossey-Bass.

Thomas, W. I., and D. W. Thomas. Situations defined as real are real in their consequences. In Stone, G. and H. Faberman, eds. 1970, *Social psychology through symbolic interactionism.* Waltham, Mass.: Xerox.

Tough, A. 1982. *Intentional Changes: A fresh approach to helping people change.* Chicago: Follett Publ. Co.

———. 1978. Major learning efforts: Recent research and future directions. *Adult Education* 28:250–263.

Vroom, V. H. 1964. *Work and motivation.* New York: Wiley.

Wergin, J. F., et al. 1988. CME and change in practice: An alternative perspective. *Journal of Continuing Education in the Health Professions* 8:147–159.

2

Curiosity

Salvatore S. Lanzilotti

It's a lot easier for me to tell you what's changed and why than it is for me
to tell you when it all began. My earliest ideas about the practice of medicine
involved a vision of myself as someone who would not only work to cure
but also work to prevent. One of the appealing things about pediatrics was
this balance between prevention and intervention. But in the real world of
practice, working in a private setting, I found a lot of my work deals with
prevention. It seems like I've always wished for more talents, more opportunity to work with children who are seriously and actuely ill. After all,
understanding my specialty involves understanding all ranges of health problems of children.

I can't say exactly when, but I got the idea that I should affiliate myself
with a university hospital in the emergency medicine department. Before I
set out to try to get a position there, I read intensively on emergency medicine
as it relates to children. I searched the literature for information on each of
the problems encountered, partly to make sure my training was up to date
but also to understand the whole field better. The more I read and the more
confident I felt, the more I wanted to have the opportunity to practice what
I had learned. About three months ago I began to deliberately pursue an
appointment, contacting the hospital's head of emergency medicine. It was
surprisingly easy since I guess it's not all that often that a well established
practitioner seeks that kind of thing. I've been affiliated with the university
hospital for a month now, and I think I have achieved some of the balance
I was seeking. The learning has continued. The patients seem to stimulate
discussions among all of us at the hospital.

CURIOSITY AND THE PROCESS OF CHANGE

The example above illustrates how pursuing personal interests can produce change. Thirty physicians described changes caused by their curiosity, their willingness or openness to pursue, expand, or develop their interests. Although the number of physicians attributing change to curiosity was relatively small, its importance as a motivation for change was evident in the types of changes that occurred, and their effects on the lives of these physicians. This chapter explores the relationship of various types of curiosity, along with other forces, to the change process. Implications for physicians, medical educators, and policy makers will be discussed.

Curiosity caused change by directing the attention of physicians toward pre-existing interests and by creating a general readiness to develop new interests. Twenty-six (87 percent) of the thirty physicians described their desire to pursue or expand a pre-existing interest, such as laser bronchoscopy, counseling patients, psychology, hypnosis, sailing, etc. The other four physicians (13 percent) reported that openness or willingness to develop new interests led to a change, for example, changing their practices to add a focus on offshore medicine, or to increase the amount of research they did by conducting clinical trials.

The role curiosity played as a condition for change varied according to the other forces interacting in their lives. For example, curiosity was either the foremost force for change, or interacted with other mutually supportive forces to affect change, or was promoted by other stimulating forces which accelerated the change process, or was triggered by a catalytic force. In all of the changes arising from curiosity, physicians reported a constellation of forces, both internal (e.g., values, beliefs, norms, self-concept, aspirations, etc.) and external (e.g., job opportunities, economic conditions, friends, and colleagues), either acting to support or prohibit pursuing an interest. The forms of the interaction of forces—dominant, mutually supportive, catalytic, and stimulating—established the conditions for change. These conditions supplied the direction and force for the change process. The process of change varied depending on the degree to which elements in the physicians' lives had to be modified, that is, through a transformation, redirection, adjustment, or accommodation. The relationship between the conditions for change and the process of change is represented in Figure 2.1.

The interplay between curiosity and other mutually supportive forces (i.e., forces which act somewhat equally and interdependently to bring about change) was responsible for nine changes (30 percent), all large and complex in nature. For example, a new interest in tandem with other mutually supportive forces caused the following large and complex changes to occur. A physician reported that he had become very active in offshore medicine, adding this new element to his private practice of fourteen years. He explained, "In some ways it was fortuitous because the opportunity arose when I was approached by a friend who asked me to become involved". One of the reasons this change occurred was

Figure 2.1
Curiosity and the Change Process

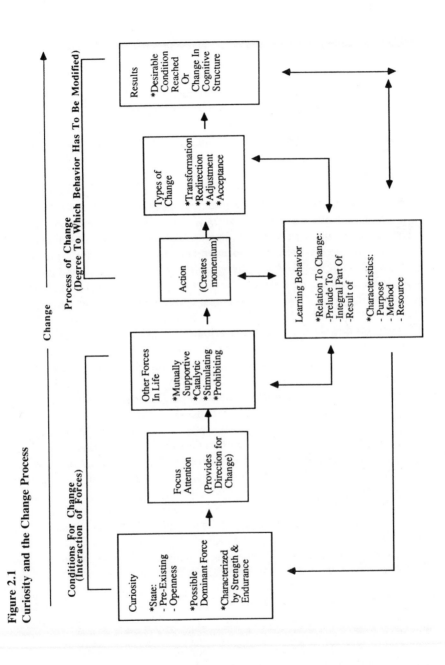

because the subject felt "an openness to change." In addition, other forces, such as the opportunity to develop an income base which included a fee for service source, and the opportunity to be involved in policy and decision making concerning health care, were important elements of the conditions for change. As a result of the synchrony of these forces, the physician decided to move in a new direction that included recruiting several of his colleagues and forming a company which now looks after workers on many offshore drilling rigs. He explained that this was a change in focus, from health care for individuals to policy and decision making in a broader sense. Finally, he reported a sense of satisfaction in being able to have an impact on the health and safety of the workers on the oil rigs, and stated that he felt "very positive about the change".

Eleven of the physicians (37 percent) described changes in which curiosity was a dominant force for a change (i.e., their interests provided the necessary impetus for change to occur). Six of these changes were adjustments, four were redirections, and one was a transformation. The following is an example of an adjustment motivated by a dominant interest. A neonatologist stated that he had been preparing to be a research scientist since his pre-med days. He pursued this interest during his residency, throughout his fellowship, and into his career in academic medicine. He enhanced the knowledge gained throughout his medical training with formal CME programs and a number of self-initiated learning projects over a period of five years. These learning projects often included many programs not directly related to neonatology. Continuous effort directed toward this interest led the doctor to discover a novel way to study maturation and development of the small intestine. Although he reported that he had to "sleep less and reduce the time allotted for recreation," he also expressed how his feelings of life satisfaction were greatly increased, for he had "fulfilled a lifetime goal." He said, "Life is more worthwhile than ever before" as he was "probing the unknown."

An additional six changes resulted from the interaction of curiosity and forces which acted as catalysts. These changes were different because, although previous interests were present, conditions were insufficient to cause any activity in pursuit of these interests. Under such circumstances, adding or subtracting an external force was necessary before these interests could be pursued. Catalytic forces in conjunction with curiosity were responsible for three redirections and three adjustments. A 35-year-old physician stated, "I see among my partners an interest in diversification. There is a need to diversify into other things besides medicine." Thus, he reported that he had felt the need to develop new interests and to broaden himself as an individual after several years of practice. He disclosed that from medical school, through residency training and board certification, the focus of the educational process, as well as the focus of his personal life, was medicine. He felt that during this period of his life his personal life had been "on the back burner." This state of mind seems to reflect the type of adaptive measures students develop in response to the stress of being in medical school. Pfeiffer (1983) cites research which suggests that students obsessed with work become somewhat "like a submarine going under, sort of like leaving the human race, only to surface at some later point after professional training is complete." It would seem that once this physician's formal training was completed, he consciously made an effort to "surface", to change his life by diversifying his activities and by pursuing interests he had previously put on hold. This effort resulted in his pursuing "knowledge for knowledge's sake" by taking classes in Spanish and business, pursuing common interests with his wife, "getting increasingly into the administrative aspects of medicine," teaching at two hospitals, developing an outside business that was not related to medicine, and spending more time among fraternal organizations.

Finally, four physicians reported changes in which external forces acted with curiosity to accelerate change. In these cases, pursuit of a pre-existing interest was already occurring but a new stimulating force was responsible for accelerating this movement. Stimulating forces were associated with three adjustments and one accommodation. An example of an accommodation brought about by curiosity and a stimulating force was described by a physician who had been working with medical students and house staff in a hospital setting for many years. Unexpectedly, he was asked to work with third-year medical students in their physical diagnosis course. He accepted the responsibility because of his belief that it is important to "provide a private practice role model instead of just the faculty role model" for medical students. The physician saw this situation as an opportunity to pursue more intensely his interest in working with students. The result, he stated, was that "it made me feel good to do something for the system." He related how he felt that he had received help from many people in his learning years at the medical school, and how he felt he "needed to put something back into the training program."

LEARNING BEHAVIOR AND THE PROCESS OF CHANGE

Physician learning behaviors seemed to occur as a condition for change, either as a prelude to initiate a change, as an integral part of a gradual change, or as a result of a change. An example of "knowing" functioning as a mutually supportive force in preparation for a change, was reported by a physician who became interested in the possibility of learning the technique of laser bronchoscopy. He used a variety of learning resources to pursue his curiosity, for example, he attended CME programs, consulted with experts, reviewed papers, viewed video tapes, and consulted with colleagues. The subject and his partners were considering whether or not this new technology would help them better serve their patients. In the last analysis, because of the costs for training and keeping skills updated, the dangers of the procedure itself, the number of patients it would serve, and the place the procedure has in the treatment process, he stopped struggling with this issue and chose not to adopt the technique. Thus, learning was a prelude to the decision. Lewin (1975) suggests that whenever a combination of forces act at the same point at the same time, there is either a locomotion in the direction of that force or a change in cognitive structure equivalent to this locomotion. In this case, a change in cognitive structure against using the technique was the equivalent of the overwhelming forces acting in that direction.

Learning that occurred as an integral part of a gradual change and, thus, as a mutually supportive force for change, was reported by a plastic surgeon who adjusted his practice over a three-year period to concentrate on maxillo-facial surgery. Although he had a pre-existing interest in this area from a fellowship he had completed, the stimulus for this change came from a patient. Once this interest had been rekindled, he began to read for theory, observe in the operating room for technical skills, enroll in CME programs that offered hands-on, practical experiences, seek information from oral surgeons, and utilize other resources such as the Cleft Palate Association. He also accepted the responsibility to direct the Cleft Lip and Palate Clinic which developed in him "a need to know more." At one point in this change, the subject organized a self-directed learning project in response to a patient with cancer of the face, who thus needed removal of a cheekbone and one eye. The surgeon stated that he did some anatomy reading, went to pathology, ordered a cadaver and performed the procedure alone, went back to more reading, and then tried to show a resident how to do the procedure on the other side of the cadaver. Once he had done this, he performed the procedure on the patient. Thus, the learning activities described by the doctor functioned as forces for change, each leading to a change in awareness and behavior, and each adding gradually to the resulting change, that is, the de facto change in the concentration of his practice.

Finally, learning that occurred as a result of a change was reported by a physician who wanted to get involved in teaching services at a hospital in which he worked. He approached the Director of Medical Education, made his request, and was subsequently assigned to a team of ten doctors who were involved in teaching family practice residents. These new duties caused him to conduct literature searches on relevant medical topics, and read the medical literature in textbooks and journal articles. In addition, he called in consultants who provided him a further opportunity for learning, especially for reviewing diagnosis on therapeutic techniques.

As is evident from the three examples above, a physician might use an assortment of learning strategies and resources, for a variety of reasons. Thus, the following analysis of physicians' learning behaviors focuses on initial learning purposes, strategies, and types of resources cited, as more important. Overall, the purpose of learning was oriented towards conceptual understanding in twenty-four cases (80 percent) and solving specific problems in only three of the cases (10 percent). In the remaining three cases (10 percent), no new learning projects were reported, as these physicians depended on previously learned information and skills to make a change. The reason for conceptually oriented learning was either: (1) to gain knowledge or to improve general skills in an area [fourteen cases (52 percent)], for example, a subject, who felt he "wasn't learning enough different things," began attending more CME meetings and became interested in learning more about arthroscopy; or (2) to gather information for the purpose of future decisions [ten cases (37 percent)], for example, the physician who was trying to decide whether or not to pursue a Masters in Public Administration degree. The strategies utilized for learning emphasized experience and interaction [seventeen cases (63 percent)]. Finally, formal learning resources were used in about half of the cases, for example, attending CME programs sponsored by the Academy of Orthopaedics; and informal resources were used in the others, for example, discussing career changes with trusted colleagues.

What is especially interesting about the learning strategies of this group is that the major purpose of learning was to improve understanding through developing or re-ordering concepts. This suggests that we must be careful not to overemphasize the prevalent assumption that adults usually have a problem-centered orientation to learning. Although the need to solve a problem can generate a need for learning, an array of forces can act as motives for learning, including one's curiosity. In addition, it is important to note that the method for learning was most often characterized by an emphasis on experience and inter-action. Discussions with colleagues, "hands-on activities," and creating situations where one could interact with others of similar interests (e.g., by actively participating in a professional organization) were learning activities of choice.

The most common constellation of learning characteristics, used by ten of the subjects, included efforts to increase conceptual understanding (purpose of learning) through experience and interaction (strategy for learning), by using informal resources (method of learning). The following is an example. A 39-year-old general practitioner reported that he had been looking for opportunities to diversify his practice and find new interests. "Charged with the decision to diversify," he met a colleague who had worked at a clinic, and who reassured him that he had the necessary skills to do this job (mutually supportive force). The physician reported that he had to find out "what it involved," that is, what skills and knowledge were required to work at a university health clinic, and "how one got into it" (conceptual orientation), before he could make a final decision. He had discussions with the colleague and with the director of the clinic (an experiential, interactive strategy). These discussions ranged over a five-month period of time. The doctor identified his colleague as the most important source of information (an informal resource). Finally, the subject decided to apply for the position in a university health clinic. The director took the request to the board who gave their consent.

CURIOSITY, ITS FUNCTION AND CHARACTERISTICS

Curiosity as a need to pursue, expand, or develop an interest spurred change in the lives of thirty physicians. Although curiosity sometimes acted as the only force for change, it often operated in consort with other forces. Changes were attributed to the interaction of a curiosity with mutually supporting, catalytic, or stimulating forces. Pursuing, expanding, or developing an interest often resulted in a major modification in physicians' lives—in addition to fifty-seven percent of the changes being major, some of the smaller changes were reported to have had important effects on career goals. For example, in one large and complex change, a physician related how she had become an activist regarding sociopolitical as well as medicopolitical and ethical issues. She reported that she had such an overwhelming interest in writing that she would spend half of her time writing on medical decision making, medical education, data analysis, medical ethics, atomic energy hazards, and cost containment in medicine. She indicated that patient care was less rewarding to her than writing. She said, ''Some people have to have their golf every week, I have to have my typewriter.''

Another indicator of the effect of curiosity was the reported increase in life satisfaction. This effect was experienced in all types of changes except small, simple accommodations. ''Specific curiosity'' (curiosity related to a particular subject and leading to specific forms of exploration) has been associated with certain characteristics such as direction of attention, duration, physiological reactivity, and verbal judgment of ''like'' or ''prefer'' (Kidd 1976). Many of these characteristics were exhibited by the physicians. Curiosity seemed to function primarily as a focus for attention, that is, it provided direction for change, either through pre-existing interests, or as a state of openness or willingness to develop a new interest (see figure 2.1). For example, statements such as ''I made a conscious decision to pursue my interest in psychiatry,'' and ''I made a decision to become more involved with clinical investigation,'' were typical of the comments describing the focus of the changes reported.

The energy generated for change by curiosity, in conjunction with other forces, was also characterized by qualities of strength and endurance. The strength of an effort to pursue an interest can be gauged by the intensity of the drive that this interest arouses. For example, the following phrases used by physicians imply the strength of their curiosity: ''I read extensively everything that might give information regarding . . . ''; ''It is the priority in my professional life;'' ''Charged with the decision to . . . ''; ''I was deeply involved in . . . ;'' and ''I felt like I was being driven . . . .''

Endurance can be assessed by the duration of exploration—the persistence of thought or action in a specific direction. In fifteen of the twenty-seven cases (56 percent), learning associated with pursuing, expanding, or developing an interest occurred over a period of one year or more, some lasting over five years. Obvious differences existed between the strength and endurance of curiosity due to several factors. First, strength and endurance seemed to be related to how important an interest was to roles such as clinician, partner, spouse, or hobbyist. Some doctors described interests that were of secondary importance, such as studying hypnosis, sailing, or reading literature from the American Medical Association, while others viewed their interests as being inextricably related to their self-concepts as physicians or persons, and highly characteristic of their work or lifestyles (e.g., changing specialty, making a breakthrough in research, or returning to school to solidify a career change).

The importance of social roles was especially evident in changes which occurred due to mutually supportive forces, as has been suggested by adult development literature (Gould 1972; Levinson et al. 1978; Havighurst 1973). In these changes (all large and complex), an interest seemed to function as a focal point for the interaction of key adult roles. For example, a 31-year-old physician with a solo practice wanted to become a parent. Consequently, she decided to organize a group practice so that her hours could be more flexible. With the help of her husband and two other female physicians, she was able to organize her life to attend to her professional and financial needs so that she could pursue her personal interests. The strength and endurance of this interest was, in part, a function of its relationship to important adult roles such as marriage and parenthood.

Another factor contributing to the differences observed in the strength and endurance of physicians' curiosity seemed to be the effective meaning associated with the interest (Lewin 1975). This meaning had a directional quality, for example, pursuing an interest might mean moving toward a desirable end in itself, or it might mean moving away from an undesirable state (being bored with one's work or feeling loss of control over one's life due to professional demands). The effective meaning given to pursuing an interest was also related to physicians' confidence, self-esteem, aspirations, or values. For example, one physician remarked that his increased learning was responsible for his "having more confidence" and "getting more respect" from cohorts.

A third factor affecting strength and endurance of curiosity was the physicians' perceptions of feasibility of success (Lewin 1975). When barriers to change were removed, or when new possibilities for change were uncovered, forces were brought to bear in the direction of pursuing interests, and the possible became the actual. Examples include one physician who was unable to pursue certain interests until after he had obtained his board certification; and another who was able to pursue his interest in curriculum development once "additional staff positions were added," thus allowing for the reduction of some of his teaching responsibilities.

Finally, the strength and endurance of many interests may have been affected by what White (1959) refers to as the "effectance urge" (by which we get satisfaction in arousing and maintaining instrumental activity that has characteristics of exploration and experimentation). He suggests that we deal with the environment by directing focal attention to some part of it, and organizing actions to have some effect on this part. Some of the changes demonstrate how pursuing an interest sometimes generated actions which developed into an almost self-perpetuating momentum for change. As physicians gathered more information to make a decision, accumulated more knowledge about an area, developed their skills in an area, or responded to new professional opportunities, they expressed a need to continue until decisions were made, competence was gained, breakthroughs were discovered, or goals were achieved. White states that the feeling of satisfaction of effectance (a feeling of efficacy) contributes significantly to feelings of interest. Kidd suggests that curiosity is not only basic to much of an individual's learning, but also to man's intellectual progress and to the advancement of science. Testimony such as "I'm enjoying breaking new ground," and "I'm enjoying probing the unknown," attests to the importance of exploring one's professional interests, both to the individual and to society.

Implications for Physicians

Physicians whose changes had the most effect on their professional or personal lives displayed persistence in pursuing their interests. A majority of the change processes lasted over a year. As one physician stated, "I have fulfilled a long-time goal." Also, physicians exhibited an inner sense of control, that is, they developed their own learning plans and created situations in which they could pursue their goals. Physicians reported organizing many kinds of learning resources, including written material, video tapes, computer technology, the use of a cadaver, formal CME programs, and colleagues and consultants, in order to learn what they wanted to know. Finally, in some cases, pursuing, expanding, or developing interests resulted in physicians experiencing greater life satisfaction and joy in learning. The satisfaction of the physician who is involved in providing health care for workers on oil rigs, or the physician whose writing has displaced medicine as a major professional and personal focus, or the joy of learning experienced by the maxillo-facial surgeon as he taught himself a procedure, are examples of the potential rewards of pursuing one's interests.

In lieu of these kinds of potential results, it seems important that other physicians ask themselves: "What would I really like to be learning about, doing, being?"; "What is prohibiting me from changing?"; "How can my friends and colleagues help me in my pursuit of change?"; "What has been the purpose of my CME endeavors?"; and "How can I rediscover the joy of learning?" Paradoxically, the first step in movement toward one's interests may be to stop and reflect, analyze, and evaluate one's present circumstances.

Implications for Medical Educators

In his research on self-directed learning, Skager (1979) suggests that curiosity can be defined in several ways, including: (1) a drive motivating all mammals which is aroused by cognitive conflict and which is reduced through exploratory behavior; (2) a personality variable responsible for such individual differences related to intelligence as observing, thinking, questioning, specific and diverse exploring, and choosing; and (3) a behavior based upon beliefs about norms, self, and goals. Accordingly, we can help students develop and clarify their interests in medicine by increasing the number of problem solving activities that promote exploratory behavior, and by decreasing the amount of lectures that promote memorization. In addition, if we want self-directed learners, we must help students develop strategies which encourage observation, questioning, decision making, and awareness and control of the cognitive processes involved in thinking (Sternberg 1985). Furthermore, in order for students to practice and develop these skills, we must establish norms in our medical schools that promote thinking, risktaking, question asking, and self-confidence. A starting point might be to ask ourselves, "What exists in our current medical school milieu that is counterproductive for learning, and to students' feelings of efficacy?"

One way to help students and physicians to pursue, expand, and develop their interests is to help them develop their ability for self-education. Based on an analysis of self-educated experts without formal training, Gibbons et al. (1980) list a number of principles that faculty can use to design strategies to help students develop self-education skills. Among others, these principles include:

1. helping learners to internalize control over their own learning;
2. integrating theoretical studies with technical training and practical application as a method of teaching;
3. helping learners generate their own drive toward their own goals rather than stimulating them to pursue goals established by others;
4. promoting, modelling, and rewarding the development of personal integrity rather than the opportunistic pursuit of offered rewards;
5. promoting originality rather than conformity, and the talents that make individuals unique rather than the tasks that make all act the same;
6. helping learners to identify themes emerging in their lives, to build on those they choose, and to create new themes they desire; and
7. creating an active environment in which learners' self-directed activities are supported and in which there are opportunities to work cooperatively with others.

If our goal is to develop the type of physician who is capable of self-education, then we must ask, "Are the principles listed above characteristic of our present medical education system?" If they are not, then it is our duty to begin teaching and supporting self-directed learning skills at all levels of medical education. The works of experts in other disciplines such as adult education (Kidd 1976; Knowles 1975; Brookfield 1984; Chene 1983; Dubin et al. 1973), professional education (Bell et al. 1983; Buchholz 1979; Barrows 1983; Harrison 1979), and general education (Lewin 1975; Beeler 1979; Scobie 1983; Perkins 1986), offer direction and guidance for accomplishing this task.

Allan, Grosswald, and Means (1984) offer some concrete suggestions to medical educators who choose to assist practicing physicians in pursuing their interests. These range from developing a user-friendly literature research system to making available formal CME activities which foster self-directed learning by supporting independent study before, during, or after a traditional program. Medical educators can also support physicians' professional learning needs by integrating formal educational programs into the practice setting, for example, the Practice Integrated Learning Sequence (PILS) program (Lanzilotti et al. 1986; Finestone et al. 1986). PILS is a practice-related, office-based CME program used by the Temple University Office of Continuing Medical Education to integrate an educational process with the actual office management of hypertension, and subsequently used in programs concerned with the diagnosis and management of refractory congestive heart failure and drug prescribing for the elderly. The participants in these programs were asked to:

1. read a monograph prepared by recognized authorities and then take a paper and pencil test;

2. apply the information to patient management in the office setting and maintain records of patient visits on a specifically designed patient report form;

3. evaluate the program and one's own learning behaviors in it (a form is supplied), and

4. submit the data generated from steps 1–3 for analysis of their performance.

As a result of the analysis (conducted through the CME office by additional recognized experts), the overall group performance was evaluated. Results were reported to all participants and recommendations for specific remedial actions were made in a second monograph.

The PILS program helps physicians pursue professional interests within a formal CME activity, allows them to take responsibility for their own learning through independent study and self-evaluation, and receive feedback on their clinical and learning behaviors, in a non-punitive climate of trust. The important element in PILS and other CME innovations suggested above is that the role of the CME provider is to help physicians pursue their interests in ways that promote a spirit of inquiry, autonomy, and self-responsibility.

Implications for Policymakers

The main task for policymakers is to devise systems that allow those working with them to meet their own needs and the needs of the people they serve. A starting point would be to assess the value teaching activity is given in the medical school environment in contrast to research and clinical activity. More rewards and awards are needed for excellence in teaching. Alternatives need to be open to faculty so that they can choose to focus on teaching rather than research, and still obtain promotion, tenure, and the respect of their colleagues. Erikson's (1963) theory of the development of the life cycle would suggest that medical schools (as part of our educational system) have a generative responsibility—"to make be" and "take care of" the next generation of doctors so that they, initially embodied as medical students, can learn to take care of others. Unfortunately, the stress generated by the traditional, predominant medical school system is not conducive to learning or teaching, nor is it very generative to those who must endure it (Pfeiffer 1983). It is hoped that policymakers will not only begin to analyze our present system but also to imagine an ideal system, one that will meet the projected needs of medical education for the twenty-first century (AAMC report 1984). To paraphrase De Bono (1985), contentment with our present "adequate" system is the biggest block there is to any search for a better alternative.

The thirty physicians who have been discussed here were motivated to learn by their own curiosity. Can we develop a medical school environment that would greatly increase the percentage of physicians who reported learning in this way? For example, what differences might we observe in physicians' learning behaviors if, as medical students, they experienced more flexibility and choice in the medical school curriculum? What would be the benefit to medical students and their career choices if medical schools were more closely associated with community hospitals, and students were exposed to patient problems from the first day and charged with the responsibility to learn medicine by solving some of these problems? In addition, how can we establish an environment that is not completely out of balance in terms of the forces interacting in students' lives, for example, interest in medicine, social life needs, financial obligations, and student obligations? As reported earlier, these forces can be either prohibitive or supportive of pursuing one's interests. How well an education system alleviates the inherent pressures of medical education and affords opportunities for exploration can be an indicator of the norms it establishes concerning support for the development of students' originality, autonomy, and independence.

Finally, policymakers can provide educational training for medical school faculty. Faculty members may be excellent academicians but they have not studied education in the way they have studied their areas of specialty. The field of education has adapted to the changes in our modern world, for example, the demand for information processing has replaced the demand for information memorizing, and teaching methods have adjusted accordingly (Sternberg 1985; Perkins 1986). If we want physicians who care for patients rather than those who treat abstract illnesses, then we must have teachers who educate the whole student as well as teach subject matter. Consequently, it is necessary that a commitment to faculty development include in-service training about how to help students explore their interests and values, develop their thinking skills (e.g., problem solving, decision making, and critical thinking), work with small groups of students (group dynamics), diagnose students' needs through questions, develop medical, problem-based learning activities, help medical students cooperate with their peers in small group learning situations, and help students design learning plans.

REFERENCES

Allan, D. M. E., S. J. Grosswald, and R. P. Means. 1984. Facilitating self-directed learning. In J. S.Green, et al., eds. *Continuing education for the health professions*. San Francisco: Jossey-Bass Publishers.

Association of American Medical Colleges. 1984. *Physicians for the twenty-first century, the GPEP Report*. Washington, D.C.: Association of American Medical Colleges.

Barrows, H. S. 1983. Problem-based, self-directed learning. *Journal of the American Medical Association* 250:22.

Beeler, K. D. 1979. How to design and conduct self-directed learning: An essential goal in education. *Kappa Delta Pi Record,* October.

Bell, D. F., and D. L. Bell. 1983. Harmonizing self-directed and teacher directed approaches to learning. *Nurse Educator,* 8:Spring.

Brookfield, S. 1984. The contribution of Eduard Lindeman to the development of theory and philosophy in adult education: A philosophical discussion. *Adult Education Quarterly,* 34(4):185–196.

Buchholz, L. M. 1979. Computer-assisted instruction for the self-directed professional learner. *Journal of Continuing Education in Nursing,* 10(1):12–14.

Chene, A. 1983. The concept of autonomy in adult education: A philosophical discussion. *Adult Education Quarterly,* 34(1):38–47.

De Bono, E. 1985. *De Bono's thinking course.* London: Ariel Books, British Broadcasting Corp.

Dubin, S. S., and M. Okun. 1973. Implications of learning theories for adult instruction. *Adult Education,* 24(1):3–19.

Erikson, E. H. 1963. *Childhood and society.* 2nd ed. New York: W. W. Norton & Co.

Finestone, A. J., et al. 1986. A practice integrated learning sequence (PILS). *Mobius* 6(1):1–5.

Gibbons, M. et al. Toward a theory of self-directed learning: A study of experts without formal training. *Journal of Humanistic Psychology,* 20(2):41–56.

Gould, R. L. 1972. The phases of adult life: A study in development psychology. *The American Journal of Psychiatry* 129(5):521–531.

Harrison, R. 1979. How to design and conduct self-directed learning experiences. *Group and Organization Studies* 3(2):149–167.

Havighurst, R. J. 1973. History of developmental psychology: Socialization and personality development through the life span. In Baltes, P. B., and W. K. Schaie, eds. *Life span developmental psychology.* New York: Academic Press.

Kidd, J. R. 1976. *How Adults Learn.* New York: Association Press.

Knowles, M. 1975. *Self-directed learning: A guide for learners and teachers.* New York: Association Press.

Lanzilotti, S. S., et al. 1986. The practice integrated learning sequence: Linking education with the practice of medicine. *Adult Education Quarterly,* 37(1):38–47.

Levinson, D. J., et al. 1978. *The Seasons of a Man's Life.* New York: Alfred A. Knopf.

Lewin, K. 1975. Behavior and development as a function of the total situation. In Cartwright, D., ed. *Field theory in social science.* Westport, Conn.: Greenwood Press.

Perkins, D. 1986. *Knowledge as design.* Hillsdale, N.J.: Lawrence Erlbaum Associates.

Pfeiffer, R. J. 1983. Early-adult development in the medical student. *Mayo Clinic Proceedings,* 58:127–134.

Scobie, R. 1983. Situational teaching: Fostering self-direction in the classroom. *Curriculum Inquiry* 13(2):132–150.

Skager, R. 1979. Self-directed learning and schooling: Identifying pertinent theories and illustrative research. *International Review of Education.* Boston, Mass.: Unesco Institute for Education.

Sternberg, R. 1985. Critical thinking: It's nature, measurement and improvement. In

Link, F. R., ed. *Essays on the intellect.* Alexandria, Va.: Association for Supervision and Curriculum Development.

White. R. W. 1959. Motivation reconsidered: The concept of competence. *Psychological Review,* 66(5):297–333.

3

The Desire for Personal Well-Being

Patricia Steen Iverson and Robert D. Fox

I've spent 20 years building my practice in OB-GYN, so it was a major change for me when I began to cut back instead. I had an MI three years ago at age 51 and I knew then that there was no way I could, or should, keep up the same sort of pace I had before. During the weeks I was off work, I spent a lot of time talking with friends and with my wife, and a lot of time just thinking. I did some reading, too, nothing specific except for several things on exercise and alternative lifestyles.

When I went back to work, I did some things differently—resigned from a couple of hospital committees, and quit the medical society's speakers' bureau, for instance. But the biggest change was scaling down my OB work and trying to schedule a full day out of the office each week to read or exercise or just spend time in family activities with my wife and the two boys still at home. I'm getting out of OB entirely now, and although I miss it, I have a better feeling about my relationship with many of the patients I'm now seeing. I have more time with them, and I enjoy it.

You know, I didn't expect anything positive to come from a heart attack at my age . . . but it did.

People make major changes in their lives as a result of such common human experiences as illness, divorce, or simply the realization with the passage of time that their personal or professional lives have not taken as satisfactory a direction as they had hoped in earlier years. This was the kind of pressure for change (illustrated in the case above) described by physicians who reacted to different personal or professional stresses, or new opportunities for betterment.

All sought to fulfill a need for a greater sense of personal well-being and life satisfaction.

The desire for personal well-being described in these cases was driven by emotions which reflected the psychological status of the physician. They ranged from hate to love, from religious zeal to ambition, and from fear and anxiety to guilt and frustration. They were internal reactions, describing a reaction to a dissonance the physician experienced between what *was* (the reality of his life at that moment), and what *should have been*—a set of expectations of self-situations which were general and diffuse in some cases rather than concrete and specific. It was this dissonance which lay at the heart of the feelings which caused change and, in many cases, learning to occur.

There were two principal ways the desire for personal well-being was manifest in the process of change. In some cases this drive for change was released by a specific precipitating event, and in others, changing was directly attributed to a growing burden of stress which eventually overwhelmed the reluctance to change. In cases where a precipitating or "triggering" event was identified, thirty-five of fifty-eight, it was most frequently viewed negatively by those who experienced it. Although in four cases of changes, the event was perceived positively (e.g. the birth of the physician's first child, or being offered an opportunity to take on a new job challenge), in the others, changing was driven by a negative view of the state of their affairs. Changing was a means to relieve the stress experienced because of personal health or life dissatisfaction. The typical statement was not, "It seemed like a fine opportunity so I . . . ", but rather, "the situation was so difficult that I . . . "

A very important kind of event that triggered the emotions causing change was a health problem experienced by the physician. In twenty-one cases, physicians had experienced heart disease, cancer, hepatitis, and other serious illness, or simply described a general malaise which they related to aging. Illness and malaise usually provoked anxiety and a drive toward a different professional or personal lifestyle. But illnesses were not the only triggers releasing the desire for personal well-being.

Events related to the physician's social situation also triggered change in some cases. These ranged from divorce, to remarriage, to pressure from a colleague or spouse to engage in recreation activities to better his or her quality of life. Also, in several cases, considerable influence was attributed to others in the physician's personal life—frequently a spouse or other relative. This was carried to the extreme in one doctor's comment, "My colleagues advised me to remarry . . . "

In those cases where no specific triggering event was evident, there was the occasional comment that, "I finally decided to do something about it. . . . " Descriptions of why change occurred suggested a slow build-up of tension and general discontent that increased over time, until barriers to change were overcome.

Changes varied according to the time between the onset of the force and the resulting change, ranging from quickly-made changes to changes made after delays of several years. Whether change occurred rapidly or after long delay was strongly related to the extent to which the problem spurring change was physical, as opposed to psychological or social. The length of time the change was delayed varied directly with the severity of the situation. Changes began almost immediately for those who found they suffered from heart disease, cancer, or other serious illness, while low-level anxiety over a history of smoking or obesity might exist for years before any change took place.

When the situation was unrelated to personal health, however, the period of delay was often lengthy. One physician was troubled because he couldn't quickly locate a clinical article or papers related to his new editorial duties. He procrastinated about his dilemma for fifteen years before developing a filing system based on an article about organizing files. Another began taking an afternoon off from his practice each week in order to engage in other, non-medical activities, a step he had been "thinking about for twenty years". As a partial explanation of these delays, some physicians described what can be viewed as "counterforces"—pressures that mitigated against change. They expressed or implied in the interviews that some of these counterforces were psychological or emotional. Positive attitudes, such as contentment with present opportunities, or satisfaction with current economic positions, moderated the pressures for change. Other, more negative emotions simply asserted opposing pressures to the pressures for change: Fear of change, guilt, fear of loss of love, and so on. Implicitly, another counterforce may have been the individual's threshold of tolerance for the tension created by distance between what *was* and what *should* be. Such tolerable discrepancies are referred to by Knox (1977) as "customary gaps."

LEARNING

Although the cause for changes discussed above was primarily the physician's emotional status, changing also involved cognition—organized, information-based thought interacting with these emotions and attitudes. Learning new information and skills was identified in thirty-three of the fifty-eight cases. Sometimes, learning served to trigger the change process. In such instances, the discontent or stress that was at the heart of the change process was released because of something new that the physician learned. The types of learning varied widely, but, in ten instances, learning was clearly a factor when formal education became the trigger for change. This occurred most often when the force for change had been present for a long time.

In other cases, learning occurred throughout the development of the emotional drive for change. In these cases, the accumulation of new information and skills was the result of increasing pressures on the physician to make a change, and may have added fuel to the efforts to change. Learning also played a role in the process of changing after the physician had made the decision to change. For example, when personal and professional stresses became great enough for one physician, he took a trip to the Far East where he studied Buddhist culture and began to make what he described as "thinking changes." The final result was a career shift from surgery to psychiatry. At other times, learning actually followed the change, as in several cases in which physicians decided to take up golfing or some other recreational activity. The decision to change in these cases often was triggered by persuasion from a spouse or friend or because of physical stresses, but after the activity was begun, learning was used to more fully integrate new ways into the physician's pattern of life.

Most frequently, after a decision to change was made, learning helped to determine the character and quality of the change. An example was the physician who found he no longer enjoyed academic work in his subspecialty, so he accepted an invitation to join a group where he was expected to handle more general internal medicine. Although he did not engage in learning related to his decision to move, after he became a part of the new group, he began to develop information and skills in some of the unfamiliar procedures to better match his new responsibilities. In a variation of this, learning was used to validate change made by a physician who followed his "gut feelings" and began to develop and use new procedures in his practice. He depended heavily on reading about successes with these procedures, so he could use them more confidently in his practice.

While education often played an important part as a catalyst for change, or as one of the factors which determined the nature of a change, this was infrequently true when a physical problem "triggered" the force for change. When change was initiated by illness, the learning which followed tended to be informal in nature. Moreover, learning projects were associated with fourteen of the twenty-one changes where physicians altered their practices or life situation by dropping or substituting some aspect (replacing some worktime with time for leisure, locating the same practice in a new area, and so on). In these cases of redirection, the decision seems to have been based on the need for change and on earlier learning, rather than on developing knowledge and skill.

When new learning was identified, very frequently both formal and informal sources were used; however, informal learning was more common overall. Learning oriented toward concrete problems also predominated, particularly in instances when the nature of the force for change, and the nature of the change, were related to personal rather than career issues. Experiential and deliberative approaches were more evenly distributed throughout the histories.

CHANGES

Although the causes of changes were attributed to a psychological or emotional state, what changed in these cases was nearly equally divided between personal life and professional life. In some cases the change was in the interaction of the physician's professional and personal life. As illustrated in the table below,

Table 3.1
Types of Consequences

Type of Consequences	Number of Cases
Professional Consequences	
Changes in practice scope/ emphasis; or attitude towards practice	16
Significant change in career goals	9
Personal Consequences	
Change in recreation/personal habits	12
Change in religious or philosophical attitudes	6
Change in marital/family obligation	3
Shift in Emphasis	
Voluntary decrease in workload/hours or in the proportion of work to leisure	12
Total	58

twenty-five of the fifty-eight changes could be identified as related primarily to professional activities, twenty-one to changes in home and family life, while twelve cases of change were described as a shift in emphasis from professional to personal concerns.

While what changed was distributed fairly evenly between professional and personal dimensions, in the twelve cases where the change was a shift in emphasis between the two, the shift was always made in the direction of the physician's personal life. In no case did the physician feel his personal happiness or well-being would be enhanced by placing greater importance on his career or spending more time in the office. In some cases this shift was triggered by an illness. Precipitating events that triggered changes were equally likely to be present whether *what* changed was personal, professional, or a balance of the two.

The types of change made most frequently were adjustments and redirections, which total eighty-one percent of the changes discussed in this chapter. Accommodations accounted for seven percent of the total, and transformation changes twelve percent. Those physicians who *accommodated*, who did as little as possible and only what was necessary in the situation, were rare (7 percent), especially when compared to the incidence of these kinds of changes in the overall study (18 percent). Such changes were described by one physician who, when he developed cataracts, responded by arranging for the surgery that subsequently permitted him to resume his normal activities; and by another who found that he enjoyed his practice more after certain developments, including an influx of new physicians, had reduced his patient load.

Adjustment changes were seen far more frequently. These physicians changed proactively but along their usual paths, altering incrementally some element of their lives or practices in response to the tensions they experienced. One who felt uncomfortable about practicing alone on his ER shifts began to share those shifts with a colleague; several others reduced commitments to hospital staff or other professional activities, or began regular exercise programs to cope with stress or illness; yet another made changes to integrate the demands of her new baby into the structure of her personal and professional life. Such changes required not only accommodation to the situation, but also taking thoughtful action to do things differently from before. However, when one considers that adjustments overall accounted for sixty-two percent of the almost 800 cases of change described in this study, adjustments made because of the need for personal well-being were relatively infrequent.

Taking a new direction by dropping, adding, or substituting a major element of life or practice was more likely to be the result of a desire for personal well-being than a result of any other force. Examples included the movement from academic medicine to private practice; the development of renewed self-esteem, and subsequent remarriage; a change from one field of medicine to another; or allowing recreational and other personal activities to assume an emphasis equal to that of career. In these cases, the action was not just to some degree different from the past, but in an opposite direction from that taken before. Overall, redirections characterized only 12.5 percent of all changes explored in this study but were the outcome in thirty-five percent of changes driven by desire for personal well-being.

Perspective transformations described by the physicians were dramatic changes in their views of the world. One physician "made a public commitment to the Lord," another decided to leave medicine and become a professional musician, and a third physician discovered a far deeper awareness of her patients as individuals following her involvement in a fatal auto accident. Each described the discovery of a new dimension in his or her life and made changes accordingly. Overall, perspective transformations accounted for only four percent of all changes studied, yet, when change was driven by personal concerns for well-being, twelve percent of changes made were large and dramatic.

Perhaps most striking is the much higher incidence of major complex changes (redirection and perspective transformations) found in these cases when compared to the study as a whole. The table below shows the proportion of each type of change found in these cases compared to the proportion of all cases in the study

Table 3.2
Types of Changes

Change Type	# in Chapter	% of Chapter	% of Total Study
Accommodation	4	7%	16%
Adjustment	26	46%	62%
Redirection	21	35%	18%
Transformation	7	12%	4%

falling into each category. When issues are personal and emotional, larger changes are more likely to result.

A comparison of changes within the chapter indicates that triggering events were no more likely to be present in one type of change than in another. However, whether or not a triggering event was present, physicians in these cases were more likely than others to respond to the force for change in their lives by moving a significant distance away from the status quo. When the psychological status was the most important force for change in these cases, it seemed to propel physicians further than was true when professional and social concerns were associated with the primary causes of change.

It is interesting that, in nearly all cases, changes were seen as complete and a sense of resolution was reached. Once such a change was initiated, whether accompanied by some triggering event or not, and regardless of the length of time the force had been in existence, the change was almost always followed through to what seemed to be a true resolution. In order to bring a change to a resolution, almost all of these physicians found it necessary to move further than simple accommodations would require, and several needed to restructure and reorient their outlooks on life or practice.

These cases tend to support the logical assumption that the physician's need for personal well-being as a psychological state is an important determinant on the way he or she practices medicine. For example, many of the physicians interviewed found a need to reduce their levels of practice, but the overall effect on patient care may well have been positive. They described better relationships with the patients they continued to see, because they were able to spend more time with them than previously. Overall, physicians felt they had achieved a better balance in their lives, and that the result was increased personal satisfaction and effectiveness.

CONCLUSIONS

In order to understand the process of change as a function of the desire for personal well-being, it is necessary to view this process from beginning to end, with an eye toward integrating the different factors and steps involved.

Prior to the decision to change, these physicians developed feelings of dissonance, because the way things "were" was not the way they "ought" to be. These feelings of dissonance were manifest in the form of an emotional and psychological state that acted as a drive, propelling the physician toward a different behavior or state of affairs. In many cases, the transition from latent to manifest was a function of a triggering event. This event was most often physical (e.g., an illness) but could also be psychological (e.g., a sudden awareness) or social (e.g., a divorce or the death of a significant person in the life of the physician). There was usually less time between the manifestation of the force and the decision to change, when the triggering force was physical rather than when it was social or psychological. However, in a significant number of changes, no triggering event was identified. Rather, the drive to change was manifest in increasingly negative feelings about the way things were. In several cases, this process of emotion-building took three years or more.

The presence of uncomfortable emotions alone was not enough, in many cases, to bring about the decision to change. Often, counterforces inhibited and moderated the intensity of the desire for well-being. In effect, these counterforces balanced the force for change for a period of time and had to be overcome before a decision to change was possible. Although counterforces were not identified in all cases, they were found to be present in an important proportion of them.

Learning played an important role in motivation to change. In many cases, learning new information was a trigger releasing the pressures to change. In others, especially those where no trigger was present, physicians often engaged in learning which appeared to augment and increase their drives to change. When the triggering event was a physical illness, however, learning played little or no role. In the process of changing, learning was a means by which the knowledge and skills necessary to make the change were developed. In this part of the change process, learning activities were not particularly different from the way that physicians learned when change was caused by other forces. There was a slight tendency for learning to be problem-oriented and for learning resources to be primarily informal rather than formal. Once again, in making the change, learning and education were viewed as less valuable when illness was the trigger releasing the change process.

In cases when the physicians' emotions and attitudes were the driving forces for change, larger and more complex changes were much more common. In fact, almost one-third of transformations and one-quarter of redirections discovered in the study were functions of the desire for personal well-being. Conversely, the tendency of physicians to simply accept and comply with the pressures for change was rare when change was driven by the desire for personal well-being. This testifies to the power of feeling as an agent of change affecting personal and professional lives.

Physicians reported that learning played an important part in the last stage of the process by validating and helping to integrate new ways of practicing and living into the ongoing patterns of their lives. Learning and education were seen as ways to improve and firm-up the fit between something new and something old. Finally, the development of something new often linked one change to the next. In fact, some physicians reported changes in chains—a new way of doing things became the triggering event for another process of change. These descriptions challenge any assumption that change is episodic and suggest that it is instead a routine and fundamental process for physicians.

An additional note about the model is appropriate at this point. In the cases of change described in this chapter, it appears that the change process is sharply attenuated when the outcome is an accommodation or a minor adjustment in practice or life patterns. It is also likely that the process is shorter when the triggering event for change is a physical problem. The change process is more likely to be extended when the triggering event is social or psychological, when there is no triggering event evident, or when the change that results is a major redirection or perspective transformation. In essence, the more concrete the triggering event, the shorter the change process. Conversely, as more major changes result, the change process is extended.

Implications for Medical Educators

Many of the physicians interviewed felt that their formal training years should have been the time to prepare for the conflicts they experienced between their personal and professional lives. One physician who blamed the failure of his marriage partly on those kinds of conflicts said that ''in medical school no one tells you'' of the toll being a doctor can exact on one's personal life. He felt preparatory courses should certainly be offered in medical school and had thought about the titles: ''Changing Life Goals'' and ''Reconciling Goals, Family, and Profession''.

Others suggested that medical students entering such a stressful profession need information about nutrition, exercise, and other aspects of maintaining their personal health. ''When teaching about stress factors and coronary disease, medical schools should relate this to the students in terms of being a physician . . . they need to learn how to take care of themselves,'' said one physician. They believed it was important to prepare students for ''life in general'' and to emphasize the value of hobbies and other ways of learning to relax.

Far from promoting a balance between professional and private life, medical training is, of course, designed to reinforce strongly the kind of single-minded devotion to work that shapes the successful medical school candidate. In view of the profession's concern about such issues as the impaired physician, however, it may be appropriate to consider medical school as the place where students can be helped to identify and resolve the kinds of conflicts that can contribute to serious problems later on.

A related factor mentioned by some was the value of making business training available to those undergraduate or resident physicians who anticipate establishing a private practice. It was felt that this would also help physicians-in-training better anticipate the nature of their future careers, while teaching time management skills important to reducing the kinds of conflicts identified in this chapter. Such opportunities to learn might also be made available at the level of graduate medical education.

Implications for CME

Although it is important to lay a foundation in the early years, the severely overcrowded medical school curriculum and the very traditional nature of medical education make it unrealistic to expect that the kinds of educational needs identified in this chapter will soon be met. Stress management, evaluating and resetting life goals, and techniques for promoting wellness within the physician's lifestyle are all issues which can be addressed for the first time, and certainly should be readdressed in CME. The mid-career physician begins to confront such issues more directly as his practice and family grow and his perspective changes. Sometimes, it is the point at which increased professional experience and confidence free him to examine issues outside his career. Health problems may begin to occur at this point as well.

The difficult issue is not only developing good teachers and presenting good information in effective ways but also making such learning acceptable to physicians who may have difficulty recognizing its availability or value. By making such learning a more acceptable means to address the stresses uncovered in this study, the hope is that fewer physicians will experience severe crises before helpful changes are made.

Information presented to the medical staff of individual hospitals may be especially helpful if the physician-hospital relationship is a strong one, as is true in many cases. Also, the local medical society might logically offer this kind of information as part of its obligation to promote the personal and physical well-being of its members. University continuing education programs may wish to offer some of this information as an integral part of some CME programs. In effect, the "student services" mission of promoting the physical, psychological, and social well-being of students should be extended to practicing physicians.

REFERENCE

Knox, A. B. 1977. *Adult development and learning: A handbook on individual growth and competence in the adult years for education in the helping professions.* San Francisco: Jossey-Bass.

4

Financial Well-Being

Richard Caplan
and Harry Gallis

I'm 58 years old and have practiced internal medicine in this city for 29 years. The major change I've noticed is that my economic status here has declined. My practice volume and income have dropped a little this past year, and I have a hunch it may continue to go down in the face of more young doctors, governmental cost-containment regulations, advertising, higher liability premiums, and competition from some of the new groups and capitation arrangements that have been developing around here.

Although I've practiced alone, I used to know all my colleagues personally, but I no longer have that kind of relationship with other doctors. Many of my older colleagues are starting to retire and I'm not getting many referrals from the new young doctors. I'm confused about this new HMO they're talking about, and I don't know what to do, or where to turn for advice. It doesn't seem like my medical school has anybody who knows what to do either . . .

The idea that financial well-being might prove to be an important force for change can come as no surprise to a thoughtful viewer of American society, with its strong tradition of economic motivation. What is new, however, is the extent to which a genuine concern, in some cases even anxiety, about financial well-being has come upon American physicians in the mid–1980s. This is not the place to analyze the phenomenon fully but simply to enumerate some of the major social trends, interrelated and rising rapidly, that account for most of what will be described in this chapter: An increasing number of practicing physicians (arising from major efforts during the last twenty years by government and educational institutions to remedy what was perceived as a great shortage); the involvement of third-party payers in the healthcare of most Americans during the past fifty years; a concerted effort by government and business to reverse what they regard as an excessive fraction of their expenditures paying for healthcare; an increasing proportion of medical services being provided by new organizational structures such as health maintenance organizations (HMO) and independent practice associations (IPA) as alternatives to the traditional fee-for-service system; the apperance and rapid growth of large for-profit institutions in the healthcare industry; and not least, the increase in malpractice actions against physicians; and other symptoms of public disaffection with the medical enterprise, considered collectively—in spite of impressive, unparalleled advances in the successful applications of bioscience to human health and disease, and the improvement, statistically speaking, in the health and longevity of the American people.

That this concern for financial well-being is new, and related to these changing socioeconomic factors, may be concluded not only by cocktail party talk or systematic interviews such as this one but also by comparing the concern for economic factors with a large survey conducted in 1980 by Denson and Manning (1982). Sixty-two percent (2,745) of their surveyed population responded to a list of twenty-six practice problems identified through a preliminary survey. Two issues that had *not* surfaced originally appeared as ''other'' responses in the completed questionnaires. One was ''a physician surplus or patient shortage in certain geographic areas or specialties'' (16/2,745 = 0.58 percent). The other was concern about ''possible competition between private physicians and HMO's'' (9/2,745 = 0.32 percent). Such a low level of concern was certainly not the case by 1985. Of further interest was the final result of their survey:

The five most frequently stated problems (government regulations of medical practice, paperwork, concern for malpractice, third-party payers, regulatory agencies) were not directly related to the care of patients. Diagnosis, therapy and the doctor-patient relationship—the essential core of medical practice—ranked respectively 24, 25 and 26 in frequency among 26 categories. Physicians thus seem to be concerned primarily by nonmedical problems. The weight of these nonmedical problems in practice may be barriers to optimal patient care by distracting physicians from the performance of their primary mission.

Many physicians feel that quality healthcare is and will be expensive; therefore, frustration arises when expenditures are cut without attention to ''quality.'' Many physicians not only face the prospect of economic insult but also, perhaps even more, experience frustration at their lack of training and understanding in the ''business'' issues of today's medical world, and their feelings that their medical and financial environment is careening out of their control. All these circumstances have resulted in an actual or feared loss of prestige, authority, freedom, and income by a group of individuals who had come to enjoy, over the past fifty years, a great amount of all four.

The physician in the opening vignette responds to these changing circumstances in large part through a sort of internal psychological adjustment (or perhaps it should be called maladjustment) but without taking much specific action beyond that. (Only 5 of 70 changes reported in this category came from women physicians.) However, not all the responses were so behaviorally passive. Among these doctors, some initiated activities that are more properly characterized as problem-solving and active rather than contemplative. These activities are definitely based much more on informal resources for learning rather than what was characterized earlier in this volume as formal resources for study. Sometimes, the effort given to learn seems small compared to the magnitude of the behavioral responses, that were occasionally large in terms of commitment of individual resources (e.g., changing the location of practice, or opening a satellite office, or joining with others to build a new clinic building). Physician colleagues, or other professionals (such as attorneys, accountants, architects, or office managers), are particularly prominent as agents to whom the physicians ventilated distress or from whom they received counsel.

Typically, the physicians in these cases read about issues of change, but they did so in a desultory manner, only occasionally settling into an organized reading effort. As mentioned earlier, formal CME, in respect to the changes in this category, was relatively low. This may be attributable to the nature of the topic but also, perhaps, to the fact that the usual purveyors of formal CME (most of which are academic institutions or professional societies) probably do not yet offer much instruction about these matters. Maybe they do not recognize fully the degree of need in this regard; perhaps they consider it inappropriate to their overall institutional mission, or possibly, they suffer a practical limitation on finding appropriate teachers for this kind of instruction. Most academic institutions and professional societies tend to seek instructors largely within their own organizations, and seldom have staff members of the type most knowledgeable and experienced to serve as teachers or counselors for the changes presented in this chapter. Also, the circumstances and problems met by individual physicians are so highly related to unique personal circumstances of location, competition, and community climate that instruction offered "in general" may be viewed as unlikely to be appropriate or adequate. The usual purveyors have tended to focus overwhelmingly on the presentation and transfer of information about biomedical science, and, at least until very recently, have tended to avoid the somewhat "tawdry affairs of the marketplace." Although academic medical centers are now forced to cope with these same problems, and make their own responses to acquire patients and dollars, their faculty members generally lack training or experience for teaching these topics.

FORCES

The increasing role of *competition* was mentioned as a major influence producing many changes. Although many remarked on the increasing number of physicians, not one of them described a role medical schools might play in response to pressures for financial well-being, or suggested that medical schools should admit fewer students or otherwise train fewer numbers. Although such a response did not appear in these interviews, articles and letters published in many recent medical and public periodicals report that such sentiment has grown in the last few years as a simplistic cure-all for geographical and specialty maldistribution.

Although many of the seventy changes evaluated in this chapter involved a clear awareness of increasing competition, definitive action was still rather slight. Two physicians were trying to learn more about alternative systems of delivery, one was considering joining an HMO, one was "fantasizing about starting a PPO," but in only three of the changes did the physician actually join one of the alternative systems. One physician had joined a physician's union.

REGULATIONS

The interviewees clearly felt bedeviled by the increasing pressure of bureaucratic *regulations* that they often regarded as either unthinking, insensitive, inappropriate, ineffective, or, in some instances, downright malevolent. A major "villain" responsible for this pressure has been the federal government, acting through regulatory effort aimed at the medical profession. An outstanding example is the recently instituted prospective payment mechanism for hospitalization, and the strong intent to expand that style of payment to cover all patient services, including physician fees as well. Many interviewed physicians feel that the paperwork and procedures obliged by these new regulations, in addition to endangering their income, are constraining, oppressive, and will adversely affect the quality of patient care. These doctors expressed concern not only for the regulatory impact on the doctor's financial status, but also considered it as a negative psychological influence on physicians, particularly their feelings about their work and their attitudes toward, and relationships with, patients and co-workers. The "climate of satisfaction" of medical work has suffered a substantial decline during the past few years.

Another force influencing financial well-being is the *aging* of the physician. The real or threatened changes in financial status, along with the change in the psychological tone of practice, have caused many physicians to consider their long range plans in a new light, including the age when they might retire from practice. Some of this response arises from chafing under growing bureaucratic regulation, and in some geographical areas and some specialities, it relates substantially to the unpleasantness and expense that hovers around the present problems of malpractice litigation and the costs of liability insurance. Therefore, age interacted with financial pressures as a force for change.

The threatening changes in the *liability* scene during recent years have caused many doctors to realize that they practice medicine more "defensively" than ever before. They dislike the intrusion of this worry into the relationships they have enjoyed with patients, and the professional choices they make about patient care. Probably, few physicians enjoy enough security about their circumstances to feel truly immune from this distress. And of course, any such discomfort translates into some modification of attitude or behavior.

Not all the changes deserved to be treated categorically; some were unique in their nature. A force that operated in one reported change was surprising: The interviewee was a radiologist who said, in effect, that she "now had too much money." Especially at her husband's urging, they had sold their "small, nice house" in a community neighborhood and bought a "lovely, large house" on a street populated by many professional offices, but with fewer neighbors or children nearby. With that change in location, they found themselves removed from friends and settings they had previously known and enjoyed. It was about a year before the considerable psychological adjustments allowed this doctor and her family to become comfortable and fulfilled in their new environment.

Financial details were not disclosed during the portion of the interviews that related to financial well-being. The interviewees always spoke vaguely about the fear of economic decline or their worries about potential loss of income. Occasionally, someone mentioned that an actual decrease had occurred, but no quantities or percentages were ever specified. In the few instances when a behavior was related to a definite decrease in income, the speaker seemed, in no case, merely to accept the decrease (possibly in exchange for a more desirable lifestyle) but, rather, tried to "work harder" by spending more hours per week, in the office, or began "moonlighting" to generate additional income, or began the effort to reorganize his practice arrangements or location. One physician mentioned his need for a greater income because of a complicated financial relationship with a bank that failed, rather than because of a decline in practice income. The circumstances necessitated that he spend more time working at the office and take fewer vacation or CME trips. In lieu of the CME trips, he settled for receiving what he considered to be very satisfactory CME through reading, discussions with colleagues, and attending talks at his local hospital, situated near a major medical center. He added that he enjoyed spending more time at work and seeing more patients.

TYPES OF CHANGES

Regarding financial well-being, the categories of change defined in this study were distributed in the following way:

Accommodation	12	(17%)	(16%)*
Adjustment	45	(64%)	(62%)
Redirection	10	(14%)	(18%)
Transformation	3	(4%)	(4%)

* = percentage for the total changes in the entire study

The distribution closely paralleled the distribution for the entire study. Thus, although a small group (17 percent) accepted change through *accommodations* (perhaps with a sigh or shrug of the shoulders), the greater number responded more actively, including fourteen percent whose response was strong enough to be considered a redirection, and four percent who experienced a more drastic transformation. To assign instances of change to particular categories is, of course, somewhat arbitrary. Agreement, among investigators, however, is good enough to identify the trends and broad patterns we seek, as discussed in Chapter 1. The overall numbers conceal a fascinating range of individual responses that can be known fully only through study of all the documents. However, some generalities seem warranted.

Adjustments tended to produce such examples as these: Opened a satellite office or moved the office nearer home or a desired clientele; worked longer hours; began to practice more defensively or modified the style of relating to patients (after realizing more fully his dependence on the way they respond to him); joined an HMO, PPO, IPA, or in one instance, a physician's union; bought a colleague's practice; sought increases in efficiency by adding computers to the business office, changed personnel, pruned operational excesses, taught office helpers how to be of greater usefulness, asked spouse to help with office work; began to advertise; took additional work as a medical examiner, emergency room physician, or government consultant; began more pre-hospitalization testing, thereby reduced the length of patients' hospital stays; acquired a new therapeutic device; obtained staff privileges at an additional hospital; or hired a marketing consultant.

Redirections were far less frequent and involved such changes as these: Joined a group, more as a defensive maneuver than as a change in philosophy about the delivery of medical services; left a group for solo practice and a greater sense of independence; found that clientele were growing older, so became less a pediatrician and more a generalist of young adults; or became a federally certified "reader" (for black-lung disease).

Transformations included three consequences among the seventy changes driven by concerns for financial well-being: Abandoned voluntary service as a teacher to devote more time to increasing practice income; changed practice from a governmentally operated community health clinic to a private practice (mostly for financial reasons, but also to reduce the burden of paperwork he felt he faced in governmental employment); or decreased his practice by fifty percent to join his wife in starting several small business enterprises.

LEARNING PATTERNS

In many instances of change, especially if categorized as accommodation, very little new learning occurred. The changes involving "feeling tone" or psychological stance more than behavior, arose from hard-to-identify reports, articles, conversations, or, perhaps, even rumors that made physicians feel uneasy or anxious about their circumstances. In such instances there was little overt response either to learn more about the issue or to "take arms against a sea of trouble." When "adjusting" involved taking an action, it tended to be more experiential than deliberative.

For those who felt enough pressure or worry about the magnitude of their practice and their income, such perturbation definitely seemed a *problem* that needed *solving* by modifying their circumstances through definite behavior; it was generally *not* a matter of "understanding" or "conceptualizing" the circumstances. This can be seen in the higher ratio of problem-solving foci to conceptual foci (2.5 to 1) for this group of changes, while a lower ratio (1.5 to 1) was calculated for all reported changes.

The kind of educational effort employed tended to be far more informal than formal. For this group of changes the ratio of formal to informal learning resources was approximately one to one, whereas, for the entire study, the ratio was approximately two and one-half to one. The informal behaviors of these physicians included, for example, discussions with accountants, attorneys, agents (from an HMO or a union), an office or group business managers, or computer consultants, and considerable reading that was relatively random rather than concerted or structured. A few individuals enrolled in a CME course, but most did not undertake new learning activities. This was especially true, of course, regarding individuals for whom the cited change represented mostly an altered "feeling tone" or attitude toward their medical work, colleagues, or patients. For example, one of the oldest physicians observed that he now had far fewer referrals. He explained that, over the years, referrals tended to be from professional colleagues who were approximately his own age; and since those colleagues had been dwindling in number as the years passed, the smaller number of them remaining in practice meant fewer referrals.

As has often been proven true throughout the history of CME, reading was a very important source of information for the physicians whose changes are discussed in this chapter. In spite of the magnitude of distress or complaint, remarkably few of these physicians seemed actually to have spent much time in a serious effort to learn about or study "the enemy." Time spent varied greatly, however. One physician estimated spending 1,200 hours working to become skilled with computers in order to use them in his office. Another physician cut his medical practice time precisely in half and devoted himself more actively to other business—all on the basis of an estimated ten hours of discussion with his wife (but who can say how much internal or "psychic time" might be devoted to making such a decision?).

DISCUSSION

This entire category of concern, financial well-being, might not have been identified at all had this survey been done earlier. All of the concerns in the seventy changes of this category relate to events in the economic climate of medical work, events (summarized at the beginning of this chapter) which have developed so recently and powerfully in the conduct of medical affairs.

Most of the reported financial changes were unquestionably associated with a negative emotional tone, and the physicians therefore adopted them with reluctance, or with grudging-to-bitter acceptance. In a few instances, the physician truly seemed to have a positive anticipatory tone (such as a small number who turned with some excitement to the addition of computers to their office, or in which a change in office location or the joining of a group seemed to elicit excitement or pleasure). On the other hand, some of those who made such a change, even obtaining a computer, considered the change painful or something that was "forced" on them; their responses were definitely defensive. This group of physicians generally seemed to have a gloomy perception of a future that promises greater competition and new kinds of practice arrangements that are either producing or threatening a decreased income. In our data base, not a single physician seemed to respond in the following manner: "Alright, I don't require such a busy practice or so much income, and I will gladly work less and earn less, but perhaps enjoy my practice and my life more." (Such a response may have surfaced among the many other changes not reviewed for this chapter.)

Implications for Physicians

Obviously, in the political and economic climate of today and tomorrow, physicians must learn about the administration of healthcare services and the financing of healthcare systems, and pay more attention to regulatory mechanisms and constraints. They must learn how to be more efficient in their work. They also should learn how to make themselves less unhappy, possibly just by spending less effort and time in grumbling and resisting the swirling changes now in progress. But thus far, ready adaptibility to change has not been an admission requirement for medical school, nor have the schools provided explicit instruction about it.

Using computers to obtain greater efficiency, and therefore protect or enhance income, seems clearly to be a component of the future. Computers alone will not eliminate deadwood and redundancy, but they could serve as part of such an effort. The expanded use of other health team members may, for some physicians or groups, promote efficiency. Physicians might devote greater attention, earlier, to planning retirement in terms of potential activities and interests as well as the fiscal aspects. They should develop alternatives for their recreation and volunteering, and perhaps even alternative sources of income, such as consulting, moonlighting, or becoming involved with business ventures that may or may not be directly related to medical or health work.

Physicians might want to study closely their lifestyles and the choices they make about many sorts of activities, in and out of medical work, to see if these choices align suitably with their values and expectations. If excesses or inefficiencies appear in their work or spare time activities, they might want to pursue some orderly pruning. A close study of one's practice, work habits, and time management, perhaps with professional consultation, might disclose ways to reduce costs or otherwise gain more efficiency. Physicians also would benefit by gathering realistic information earlier in their careers, to help plan for the fiscal and psychological aspects of retirement. They could plan life trajectories that move them, as they age, to positions that pay less, but require less time and responsibility.

Unless some radical event disturbs the present path of medical work and the attitudes of government and the public, advertising and marketing for the individual physician and medical group are here to stay. Therefore, to prescribe study, reflection, and ultimately action on these matters, seems warranted; to follow the prescription seems wise.

Implications for Medical Educators

Throughout the medical education continuum, but especially at more advanced levels, teachers need to provide more instruction that deals with: Computers and their many potential uses beyond word processing; practice efficiency; cost containment, especially learning to weigh cost-risk-benefit ratios realistically, to avoid the urge to order and do everything that might conceivably be done to or for every patient; marketing and advertising; office management; and techniques for coping emotionally with the stress of competition and the many things that "doctoring" did not formerly involve. Learners at all levels need to grow more comfortable about sharing information without feeling defensive or threatened. Admittedly, that was far less difficult in an era when competition seemed less direct and forceful than it has grown to be in the last few years. Also, educators should attend to the many ethical considerations that relate to providing quality medical service in the face of the many pressures to contain costs by cutting corners.

Medical educators need to recognize, more fully and consciously than they have during much of the last thirty years, that the delivery of healthcare, to individuals and to society in general, includes far more than simply the delivery of biomedical science and techniques. Additionally, since healthcare requires much know-how about both individuals and diverse groups, healthcare educators should give much more attention to the psychological, sociological, anthropological, legal, and religious structures, among other needs of society.

Implications for Policymakers

Cost containment incentives that are driven mainly by dollars and the "bottom line mentality" may grievously damage the attitude of the medical profession in its relationships with patients, and in its efforts to provide quality medical services. The sense of trust and covenant, developed over millenia in behalf of the profession's healing ability, is fragile. If ravished, it will not easily recover.

Policymakers might help stimulate alternative rewards for healthcare providers so that dollars alone would play a less salient role as each builds his or her sense of personal status. Mechanisms to help restore a sense of learned professionalism would be welcome, along with mechanisms to provide accountability, less burdened by administrative clutter. For example, policymakers could contribute greatly through their crucial activities that channel support to research, which, more than any other factor, promises to help health professionals improve their therapeutic efficacy. The great majority of individuals who entered medicine, and continued in it, probably did so with a genuine urge to help people get well and stay well. Rarely has altruism been totally evaporated by the passion to become wealthy. If physicians can be more helpful to patients, the gratification attained may somewhat replace the more material rewards.

Speaking at a 1983 conference, Altman (1986, 44) reluctantly concluded "that economic issues have a greater influence on physicians' pattern of practice than they are willing to admit, and the changes in these patterns occur much more rapidly in response to economic pressures than to scientific realizations." If he is correct, physicians, educators, and policymakers all need to address the effect on physician behavior and health outcomes, produced by a working climate in which corporate medicine grows increasingly dominant, and society is indecisive in its policies about medical indigency, thereby placing physicians in an awkward and tense situation between their own well-being and that of their patients. The present turmoil in the arena of medical economics, generating physician anxiety and dissatisfaction, will surely produce long-term, baleful effects in patients and society. Recognition of this problem will provide the first step toward a remedy.

REFERENCES

Altman, M. 1986. In Allen, A. S., ed. 1986. *New options, new dilemmas*. Lexington, Mass.: Lexington Books.

Denson, T. A., and P. R. Manning. 1982. Current problems in medical practice as viewed by California physicians. *West Journal Medical* 136:369–372.

5

Stage of Career

Nancy L. Bennett
and Martyn O. Hotvedt

The patients are mine and no one else's. I now have the ultimate and final responsibility. At first, I was a little scared because I feel much more on my own than I used to. Now I have to look for answers myself. While I was training, I acted as if I was on my own, but I always knew the faculty were there. Things are slow, but I think a practice is sort of like building a house—one brick at a time. I'll feel more secure about how I practice, what I need to know, how to make decisions, and what my job will be like after more experience . . .

I want to get out before they kick me out, although I'm probably a better physician now than I have ever been. It's natural to age, but I have begun to ask myself where I am and what I am going to do with the rest of my life. I am being phased out by fate—sometimes I think patients are guessing I will retire soon, so they don't want to start care of a newborn here and then have to change physicians before the child reaches adolescence. I don't see as many babies as I used to, and I work more with adolescents. All in all, I have become very aware of my age and the passage of time. But I don't know if retirement is the best thing for me yet.

For physicians, the predictable changes of adulthood are not exactly "right." From the beginning, perhaps because of long years of training, many feel they start off-schedule in their own professional development, and the feedback they receive does not involve many of the same signals found in some other professions. Job titles and tasks usually do not change, and the sense of starting out late may demand a sense of catch-up. The stories of the physicians in this chapter

(59 cases) suggest that the kinds of changes they make, and the learning they pursue to make these changes, are directly tied to stages of career development. Further, given the stages, there is tension in correlating the intensity of their development in medicine with the other aspects of their lives.

Many predictable changes are age-related. Completion of schooling, marriage, and a first job are usually expected to occur at certain ages (Knox, 1977). The physicians to whom we spoke talked about three stages in the development of their careers: The first was a time to gain entry into the practice of medicine; the second, a time to develop and establish a distinct place for themselves; and the third, a period of pressure to relinquish that place. Although each of these stages and their effects were modified by individual goals and by the way personal, professional, and societal pressures were perceived, their descriptions of each stage contained a set of common concerns and traits. For physicians in this study, the length of time associated with the first and last stages of their careers was fairly short and seemed to contain relatively few options. Their responses, as a group, were more uniform and more predictable. The middle stage was longer and less uniform.

"Breaking in," the first stage, was associated with setting up a practice of medicine and occupying the roles of a new physician. With a new practice came all the adjustments and changes necessary to continue careers. Those "breaking in" spoke of pressure to become established and make up for time lost through extensive schooling and training. Ten cases described changes associated with "breaking in." Nine of the ten physicians in this group described how they acted on their decisions to enter into practice. Most were interested in becoming part of the medical establishment, and were concerned with finding a job to fit into the medical community. This step marked the beginning of postgraduate professional development. After years of "practicing" in school, the experience was now "real." Now was the time to reconcile earlier expectations with reality, a process usually plagued by conflicts.

Changes associated with "breaking in" were attempts to resolve internal conflicts about the need for good work situations, for trust in themselves as physicians, for increased independence and responsibility, and for further definition of their relationships to patients. Although most faced and dealt with these pressures, one physician interviewed had difficulty accepting the role of physician. She expressed serious conflicts relating to both the medical system and to her dislike for direct patient care. Her reaction was to explore alternative medical care systems and a medical role that did not directly include patient care. One of her emerging ideas was to work in the development of computer systems for medical care. The change she made demonstrated one quite unusual reaction to the pressures and traditional expectations for physicians "breaking in."

Another physician, in setting up practice, began to rely less on diagnostic protocols learned during training and, consequently, completely reformulated her ideas about treating patients in her office. She described a newfound willingness to trust herself in ways that were unacceptable to her mentor during residency training. This caused the perception of an even stronger obligation on her part to "be sure" of her course of action. She spoke of the ongoing struggle and the tension associated with this change, that she felt impinged on all areas of her practice, including her relationships with partners, other peers, and patients. A new idea about her professional behavior was beginning to take shape as she "tried on" her version of the "established physician" role.

Those "breaking in" were quite similar to one another in their concerns. All expressed a need to establish a position for themselves in the medical care system. The changes caused by "breaking in" were most often incremental. Behavior was being tailored to fit each role and each situation, usually with stress and effort. However, not all physicians attempted to design a traditional physician role. Concern for other roles in life was obvious.

The second developmental stage focused on the process of "fitting in"— finding a place in medicine that reflected the characteristics of the physician both as a unique professional and a person. It was a period of confusion and questioning about how to fit into medicine, and how to fit medicine into broader life. Twenty-six cases described changes associated with "fitting in."

The physicians who were "fitting in" were more likely than those "breaking in" to describe either small, simple changes or large, complex, dramatic changes in response to the pressures of this middle stage. Both career and personal "clocks" were evident as many physicians expressed a sense of concern for staying "on time" or for using the "time left," rather than referring to their futures as unbounded. There were also references to a growing introspection about the role of medicine in one's life and the vagueness of boundaries separating the role of physician from other roles. The twenty-six changes described by physicians "fitting in" fell into four areas: Daily medical practices, professional goals, professional affiliations, and the relationship of medical roles to other roles.

Nine physicians described changes in the characteristics of their daily practices. Included were changes in patient population, new patient problems, work patterns (such as altered consulting arrangements), and personal aspirations (such as pulling back from the lead in the creation of a new department). Two physicians intentionally altered daily practice as a result of a combination of experience and introspection, attributing the changes to their clear visions about the way they preferred to practice medicine. One concluded that increasing the time spent on taking histories allowed better and more efficient medical management, while another expressed less need to firmly establish a diagnosis before beginning treatment. Both were departures from practice patterns developed while "breaking in."

Seven doctors altered their professional goals. Two of these shifted their emphasis from practice to research, while another decided to be less involved in new research efforts because he felt that his age (52) precluded long term commitments. One physician, who was 43 years old, completely redirected his research, commuting several days each week to a distant center to intensively study a new technique, while reducing time in his current position to accommodate the major time commitment for the new project. In retrospect, he described this as a result of a mid-life assessment of the way his current work matched his ideal worklife. He decided it was necessary to think through his real and ideal accomplishments to develop new, more appropriate goals. One physician discussed an unhappy sense of having reached all of his initial goals by his early forties, wondering what to do without further direction for his life.

Two physicians dramatically transformed their situations. The first sold his large urban practice, moved to a distant site, and bought part of a small practice in order to write a book. He described this as the resolution of an intense mid-life questioning of purpose that resulted in a new set of personal and professional expectations and goals. The second physician transformed his ideas about terminal illness because of his experience with his mother's illness and death, and the role he had played in the care of a dying colleague. He described this as a major restructuring not only of the way he thought and acted toward the dying, but also his feelings about patients' control of their surroundings during palliative care.

Changes in board certification status and professional affiliations were discussed, since the middle years are an important time to become involved in professional activities. Board certification was achieved by two physicians, one after a previously failed attempt. Two physicians altered professional group memberships, one by becoming more involved, and the other by dropping out of a professional group in which he played a major leadership role. Both were in their early forties.

Seven doctors described how their medical roles had changed as a result of the age related conflicts between work and other roles and responsibilities. This was especially evident among women, who described major changes that allowed time for more attention to their roles as parents.

Among the twenty-six physicians "fitting in," the largest number reacted to change by making adjustments, followed by those who simply accepted whatever changes were required. The third largest number of cases involved physicians who described a redirection of their lives and practices in response to their developmental stages. Although the ages of those making changes to "fit in" ranged from thirty to sixty, the majority of those making major changes were between thirty-nine and forty-eight, findings consistent with the more dramatic changes that may occur in this transitional period.

The third stage, "getting out," refers to events and situations which tend to lead toward reduced involvement in medical practice and, eventually, to retirement. During this period, physicians reported high levels of awareness of their ages and the time they had remaining. The effects of this awareness included changes in their estimates of their own health, their professional standings, their views of the world, and the world's view of them as "aging physicians."

Most of the comments of twenty-three physicians "getting out" reflected their intense concerns and sense of internal conflicts. In all of these, the source of concern was the sense of their ages, but other forces were also mentioned. Only one physician talked directly about an association between age and medical competence. However, several believed that others were concerned about his or her competence. Four physicians described some of the conflicts experienced by this group from different perspectives. One physician vividly described the clash of slowing down with his lifelong drive to continually improve his abilities as an obstacle to his retirement and a source of much conflict about "getting out." A surgeon, who described the negative stereotypes of aging as opposed to real ability when learning new procedures, now finds it necessary to apologize for being fifty-seven instead of thirty-five. Ironically, a third physician, who was beginning to "feel older," sat on a board that attempts to stop older physicians from operating because of their deteriorating abilities. He said he felt it necessary to "get out" due to his gut reaction not to push his own luck. Finally, one physician said he wanted to "get out" before they asked him to "get out," although he was a better physician than ever before. These examples, which characterize the "getting out" stage of the "clock," illustrate a perception of discrimination based on age instead of competency.

Financial planning was a major concern, as was the desire for shorter workdays to allow more free time. Some of the relatively younger physicians in this older group also talked about the long-term physical stresses of practice and the pressures of outside regulation as forces that contributed to change. One physician talked about his unusual plan to work for three months each year and to sail for the other nine months. More frequently, physicians spoke of nearing "retirement age," and thinking about options. There was a clear expression of the need to begin making changes in practice patterns far in advance of retirement because obligations to patients, peers, and hospitals had usually been made over long periods and were difficult to relinquish.

Thirteen physicians were actively planning retirement. Six wanted to retire to escape rigid schedules or heavy workloads, or to spend time with family and other interests. Four felt they were being forced to plan retirement by changes in patient populations, general increases in malpractice risks, or the social stigma of being an "older physician." One restructured his life to allow compilation of a major multivolume work covering a large segment of his field of practice. He poetically described this work as the culmination of his lifelong dream of contributing to the field of medicine, which had contributed so much to his life. At seventy-six, one surgeon had stopped performing surgery but continued to consult in his field, with no plans to retire.

The physicians who were "getting out" ranged from forty-seven to seventy-six years old. The group was marked by concern for the future in terms of financial security and professional self-worth. Estimates of competence in practice situations were usually voiced second to personal concerns. In our study, slightly more than one of three physicians over sixty-five described a change driven by pressures to "get out of practice."

LEARNING

Learning, as part of change, is linked to age and stage of career. For most of the cases (86 percent), learning was essential. All those "breaking in" used learning as a part of change. However, among changes made by those "fitting in," learning was used differently in the change process. When small changes were made, learning was used in only half of the changes. When practices or ways of life were adjusted in modest ways, or altered in major ways, all but one change involved learning. All but two of the changes precipitated by pressures for "getting out" required learning. Both were small and simple acts of acquiescence.

Two characteristics of the learning process for these physicians stand out. First, learning through experiential activities decreased with age and career stage. The majority of cases of change, (60 percent) for those "breaking in," relied on experience. Experiential learning dropped to approximately half of those "fitting in," and to one-third of those "getting out." Deliberative learning activities that emphasized reflection over direct experiences increased with age—two-thirds of those "getting out," as opposed to less than half (40 percent) of those "breaking in," emphasized reflection in their learning strategies. Second, intentions to solve specific problems, as opposed to intentions to gain a conceptual understanding, were more important to those "breaking in" (60 percent) but of less interest for those "getting out" (19 percent). Those "breaking in" showed a slight preference for learning from informal resources (60 percent), usually colleagues.

How these physicians learned was influenced by their ages and stages of professional development. Learning from informal sources and experiences, for the purpose of solving a specific problem, was associated with half the changes of those "breaking in" but was less evident in changes of those "fitting in" or "getting out." On the other hand, deliberative efforts directed toward a better understanding on a conceptual level was used in only twenty percent of the changes of those "breaking in," versus sixty-two percent of changes associated with "getting out." Conceptual understanding, using formal resources, was not often sought by those "breaking in" (20 percent), but was used by approximately half of those "getting out."

The power of traditional medical teaching, especially for those "getting out," may help to account for more emphasis on deliberative strategies and formal resources. The desire to be part of the mainstream and conform to what they believed to be the local medical community's standard practices, coupled with a lack of experience, may account for the focus on specific problems by those "breaking in." Conversely, the greater emphasis on concepts and general understanding by those "getting out" may reflect a mix of experience with interests in broader issues. Based on their stories of change, this broadening of perspective was certainly part of their efforts to reconcile advancing age with demands of professional practices and personal lives. The pattern of growing emphasis on conceptual learning, over time, seems consistent with the idea of incorporating experience into a broader and deeper understanding characteristic of maturation.

Those simply accepting changes (14 cases) most often used more informal resources for learning. However, almost half of those who described these small changes provided no information about any new learning as part of the change process. These small changes without new learning activities accounted for seventy-five percent of all changes made without any reported efforts to learn.

Adjustments (32 cases) in behavior or performance were most often accomplished through attempts to understand or conceptualize an issue, as opposed to attempting to solve a specific, concrete problem. This was especially true for all but those "breaking in." About one-third of those who made adjustments in their lifes or practices described a school-like approach, depending more heavily on formal resources, and deliberative strategies, to understand issues.

Change processes which resulted in redirections (9 cases) or transformations (4 cases) of the structures of lives and practices were more often characterized by attempts to conceptualize an issue rather than looking for answers to specific problems. For the few cases of transformation, experience was the primary strategy for learning.

CONCLUSIONS AND DISCUSSION

Physicians are trained with a sense of the "right" action at the "right" time, a mandate which applies to both their professional and personal lives. In this study, the physicians' personal identities with career were intense, and few talked about aspects of their lives that were free of the influence of their practices. They described three stages that seemed to demand change and forced ideas about how to practice medicine—"breaking in," "fitting in," and "getting out." Physicians "breaking in" to the medical care system most often accommodated or adjusted to the pressures surrounding the move from training to clinical practice. New roles were adopted, some with effort and stress, as those "breaking in" most often concentrated on becoming part of the system. Overall, the physicians in this group perceived relatively few options, but many mandates for change. Because "desirable" new positions were thought to be scarce, new practitioners felt that the long-term consequences of their decisions were many, and that it was critical to break into the mainstream by attending to the protocols and the practice preferences of peers already in practice. Medical community standards were important.

Those "fitting in" described not only wider variation in types of change but also more dramatic change. Simply accommodating to necessary changes was more common, but there were also more complex redirections or transformations. The need to reassess lives and to "fit in" usually began about three to five years after entering into practice. Physicians used experience to develop a sense of how they wanted to practice medicine and to live. Interpretations of change were both positive and negative, as some viewed change as adding to their lives and others as detracting. Their concerns were varied, with few common threads, and with a large variety of possible professional and personal directions. Physicians developed more uniqueness as changing professional and personal lives were measured against previous personal and professional ideals.

The physicians "getting out" seemed more like those "breaking in," in that they perceived fewer options and more mandates circumscribing their professional and personal lives. Thinking about relinquishing professional roles through retirement was stressful. Societal concerns were sometimes in conflict with self-assessments. Institutional age restrictions posed more as limits for practice than measures of competence. The entrepreneurial aspects of private practice with high autonomy were viewed by those "getting out" as threatened by, and conflicting with efforts of others to control their practices. Some physicians felt forced to leave professional obligations before the time was "right."

When, over time, changes in career are added to changes in personal lives, physicians may experience different stages in different aspects of their lives. For example, professional life may move forward, and personal life may lag as attention is diverted from marriage or parenting to developing professional skills and opportunities. Or, professional progress may be temporarily slowed to allow time for family or personal interests. Development in one dimension did not necessarily predict the same growth in another. To move from the point at which an old stage of life was viewed as inappropriate, but a new stage was not yet defined, required time and effort. The transition points associated with each stage of life were clearly and vividly described as demanding, stressful, and a difficult bridge.

Learning was an important mechanism for change. Its nature seemed to be shaped, in part, by the extensive traditional schooling physicians experience. Understanding a problem was more often based on developing clear concepts through help from formal or approved sources, rather than based on gaining solutions to specific problems through direct experience. This seemed especially evident for the older group, who were educated when concepts, more likely than problems, were the overriding concerns of medical instruction. On the other hand, the tendency to be problem-oriented, and to use experiential learning strategies and more informal learning resources was more common in younger physicians, particularly when the issue was nonclinical.

Although, occasionally, changes of all types were made without reports of new learning, they were most common when change was a simple accommodation. When learning associated with accepting these minor changes did occur, informal resources predominated.

There are several ways that conclusions about changes in physicians' lives and practices attributed to age and stage of career may be integrated with the other valuable perspectives on development in adulthood. Levinson et al. (1978) described adult development as a succession of seasons, each with a qualitative difference and distinctive character. The "life course has a certain shape that evolves through a series of definable forms. No season is better or more important than the other. Each has its necessary place and contributes its special character to the whole." Levinson defines ten periods and transitions.

The first two periods encourage people to move into the adult world (17–22 years old), or establish a home base (23–28 years old). A transition point (29–32 years old) creates a sense that "real" choices are being made. To this point, physicians who have been in school and training may lag behind most other professions entering the adult world. Medical students experience a step-by-step progress through school. College and medical school are followed by three to six years, or more, of postgraduate clinical training. Because excellence in schooling is mandated, many must concentrate on learning and grades to the relative exclusion of other social activities or personal development concerns. Through training, physicians may retain some characteristics of pre-adults which retard the "career clock" compared to that of peers in other fields. Yet the long schooling in medicine creates a very strong sense of "proper" timing by focusing on appropriate status and achievement as physicians develop. The move from training to practice initiates the first of the three stages in the development of physicians as described in this chapter.

The next four periods of Levinson's seasons of life map the middle years. People settle down (33–39 years old), investing their time in what has become more important, often work, family, and community. As that process is completed, a time to reassess and question life begins (40–45 years old). It is followed by a period of resolution (46–50 years old) in which creativity may either decline or be enhanced. The transition of the early fifties (50–55 years old) typifies middle adulthood for many.

For physicians, these middle periods may be the time for establishing and refining their professional lives. However, the sense of entering early adulthood at a relatively late age may induce a sense of urgency about "pushing ahead." This sense may be compounded by the intense demands placed on physicians to remain up-to-date in their practices. Personal life may also have developed on a delayed schedule and may also create a sense of need to "catch up." All of the urgency may make the reassessment and questioning that is typical during the middle years particularly intense for physicians.

In Levinson's terms, the final three periods of the adult lifespan build the second part of middle adult life (56–59 years old), conclude it (61–65 years old), and begin preparation for late adulthood (65 + years old). These stages precipitate a time of intense conflict for many doctors. Self-assessment of competence begins to conflict with age-related social expectations. For example, hospitals may impose age restrictions for physicians admitting patients, or patients may begin to look at practitioners in their sixties as "older." As referrals go to younger doctors, intentions to maintain a high level of professional practice in the middle years may go unrewarded. Physicians' patients may view new procedures and new technologies as if they were the domain of younger physicians whose training is more current.

Age norms and age expectations are in the words of Neugarten (1964), "prods and brakes upon behavior.'' Men and women are not only aware of the ''clocks'' that operate in various areas of their lives, but are also aware of where they are in regard to these ''clocks.'' Consequently, they readily describe themselves as ''early,'' ''late,'' or ''on-time'' with regard to family and occupational events. For example, men perceived a close relationship between their ages and their careers; middle age is a time to reassess achievements in terms of being ''on-time'' or ''late.'' Physicians in this study often referred to themselves in terms of time when describing specific forces or changes: ''It's late to be making a major change in research''; or ''It's time for me to be more involved in my professional society.''

Implications for CME

The stages of development portrayed in these cases imply that physicians change their ideas, over time, about how to practice medicine. Changes may be small or large and may apply to medicine as a whole or to individual parts of a single practice. Further, as physicians age in their careers, they appear to change their ideas about the place of medicine in their lives. CME may be used differently according to career development stage. Physicians ''breaking in,'' for example, may use CME as one way to establish for themselves the local and national norms used for practice by peers and experts. Most physicians ''breaking in'' wish to fit into the mainstream of the local group, preferring not to deviate from local norms. Medical educators may see those ''breaking in'' attending programs because they wish to know about local practice, hear influential local practitioners, discuss community protocols, and make known to the professional community the current state of their own training and expertise. In medical practice, the desire to demonstrate the current state of training may result in a practice that heavily utilizes ''new,'' ''innovative'' procedures to stress emerging expertise to peers and patients, while attempting to abide by local ways and means. Participation in CME may emphasize the confirmation of what is already known, or the adaptation of training to current circumstances. New procedures already covered in training may be of lesser interest. Those ''breaking in'' may be particularly interested in CME more as a way of becoming a member of the professional community, rather than as a way to learn a new procedure.

After their places in medicine are established, physicians ''fitting in'' to the system may intensively search through CME for techniques or concepts appropriate for each's emerging expertise and practical experience. They may begin to diverge from locally acceptable ways to test other ways. Further specialization may begin as practice volume, local opinion, and personal interests develop. Some may seek change, for example, to allow restructuring a practice pattern to emphasize a specific area of expertise or interest, or to provide better scheduling. For some, technical skills may be less central, with the focus replaced by administrative concerns or more global views of issues. Others ''fitting in'' may wish to decrease or change the format of their CME participation due to competing interests of family or community roles. Also, membership in a group may be a deciding factor for the source of CME used in patient care. For example, the American Cancer Society recommends screening procedures. Those recommendations are different from the recommendations of the American College of Obstetrics and Gynecology and other groups. Membership in, or allegiance to, one or the other may dictate how a group of patients are screened and which peers are used for reference. While there is not a "right" answer for many health issues, the differences among acceptable answers may be significant. Practice in a prepaid healthcare setting may also result in significant differences in ambulatory care.

In contrast to physicians "breaking in," those "fitting in" may use CME as they become more interested in new procedures to update training. They may begin to further refine an area of interest and expertise to create a personal specialty. Experts from outside the local area may provide a broader range of ideas or a new comparison with actual experiences. Increased financial security may allow broader travel and more options for education. A group of those "fitting in" may have difficulty in finding the place for medicine in their lives. Professional roles may influence or be influenced by marriage or divorce, having or not having children, and becoming involved in church or community roles. Alcohol or drugs may become an influence. Others may devote all their energies to medicine. Some may be unable to "fit in," potentially resulting in stagnation, a downward slide, or a move out of the field. These people may not participate in CME or any other form of education.

As physicians begin to think about "getting out" of medicine, concerns for professional control and image may be critical. "Getting out" may be perceived as mandated before the time is "right." They may wish to be seen by the professional community as actively educating themselves, fully integrated into the mainstream of medicine. Physicians concerned with timing their withdrawals from practice may become interested in self-assessment of practice management to gain a measure of reassurance about their competence. Legal concerns may become increasingly worrisome, in that any major lawsuit may remove financial security at a time when income potential is decreasing. Some may return to or stay in the traditional CME system to maintain contacts and reputations. A small group of those "getting out" have the potential to move to a more global perspective, becoming active as spokespersons or elder statespersons.

The richness of these data on changes driven by age and stage of career, while impressive, only begin to provide clues needed for a fuller explanation. The concept of self-change evolves over time. Certainly, physicians assess their personal and professional selves in individual situations, in terms of their individual goals. But, as a group, they talk about their professional and personal changes in a way that is consistent with Levinson's view of the seasons of life. For example, the sense of control over their development shifted dramatically. Those "breaking in" and "getting out" felt "owned" by the medical system. There seemed to be few options and many mandates. Those "fitting in" described more of a sense of freedom or personal ownership of the direction of their development. The transition between "breaking in" and "fitting in" may be, in part, a shift from perceiving few options, with little control, to one of perceiving many options with much greater personal control. However, the transition between "fitting in" and "getting out" seems to reflect some loss of this personal control and a return to fewer options.

The practice of medicine, unlike most other occupations, does not exist within a formal organization with a clear authority hierarchy, job descriptions, and lines of advancement. Job titles do not change as expertise, influence, and experience expand. Promotions, with new titles, are not directly acquired by an individual as an acclamation from his or her superiors. The cues for status are therefore different. In medicine, the role of peers is especially critical in determining one's place in the structure of the profession. The movement through career stages, as a result, may be subtle, and felt indirectly by feedback from peers and patients as well as by self-assessment.

Because the role of peers is so important, it is interesting to hypothesize the effect of career development on professional relationships. Each individual physician is at a certain stage of development, while other colleagues are at different stages. Components of satisfying relationships, differences in styles of relationships, or even conflict, may be influenced by the match of career stages with all the ramifications, for example, of changing views of medicine, perceived number of options for practice, and stage of other roles in life. Perhaps a sense of being "out of synch" relates to the match in stages. On the other hand, perhaps a version of mentoring or a wider perspective is gained by there being other physicians in the same match of stages. Style and type of training might be superimposed on these relationships to understand more fully the dynamics of peer relationships.

These descriptions of change begin to elicit ideas for other important questions. For example, of the proposed stages, "fitting in" is the longest and most diverse. What is required to "fit in?" The process of "fitting in" might, for example, include settling down, branching out, "narrowing in," singularly, or in some combination. How do the "elder statespersons" and distinguished practitioners develop? Are these people who are able to complete all the tasks of a given stage before they begin to work on the next stage? Levinson describes the need to resolve issues and complete tasks at each developmental period in order to move forward. Perhaps these are the examples of such people in medicine.

Disaffection is a topic discussed with relish, intensity, and concern. A case can be made for career disaffection most readily becoming obvious during "fitting in." With some sense of security about establishing a place in medicine, physicians begin to determine more exactly how they wish to look for the perfect way to practice medicine. That process may be triggered, for example, by increasing satisfaction, mounting frustration, or waning interest in practice. On the other hand, school/training burnout would seem most predictable during the "breaking in" stage. The long years of study may have taken a toll which becomes especially obvious when the energy to make a major transition is not readily forthcoming. "Getting out" may include depression or frustration that results from the lack of external reward for staying up to date, and practicing thoughtful medicine based on years of experience. These data are not sufficient to detail the stages, and more directed study is needed.

From another view, the careers of physicians seem well regulated. Those "breaking in" and "fitting in" describe a sense of being fully, but indirectly, regulated by a career "clock" and a sense of what should be done at a certain stage. But, rather abruptly, society enters the scene to exercise a "strong arm" on those nearing the "getting out" stage. Physicians perceive this in their own assessments of physical status, others' views of "older" physicians, and discussions about mandatory retirement. If socialization into the role of physician begins with medical school and predicts much about those "breaking in," is there a "desocialization" from the role of physician for those "getting out?" Does this process predict the postdoctoring years? The status of "older physicians" and of those "getting out" is glossed over in medicine as it is in most other occupations. It is important for future investigations to include this topic.

REFERENCES

Knox, A. B. 1977. *Adult development and learning*. San Francisco: Jossey-Bass.

Levinson, D. J., et al. 1978. *The Seasons of a Man's Life*. New York: Alfred A. Knopf.

Neugarten, B. L., and Associates, eds. 1964. *Personality in middle and late life*. New York: Atherton Press.

6

Competence

R. Wayne Putnam
and M. Donald Campbell

For many years I used to be unhappy with my acromioplasties. Because the end results did not justify the procedure, I switched to nonoperative management. However, three years ago my partner attended an orthopedic academy meeting and learned about a new procedure that led to improved results. He discussed it with our group on his return, and so the next year I went to the meeting specifically to seek information on this procedure. I attended three formal lectures and discussed the differences from previous techniques with other attendees at the meeting. On my return I discussed it with my own partners and then did approximately ten hours reading about the procedure in orthopedic journals. When the first appropriate patient came along, I had no difficulty with the procedure, and my partners began using the new technique as well. We continually discussed our findings and results. The improved outcome from the new procedure gives me a good feeling of being more competent in handling such a problem. I subsequently made an improvement to the procedure by modifying the technique slightly to suit myself.

''Doing one's best'' in the middle of an explosion of knowledge can be a tough job. Like others, physicians strive to practice their profession in a way which meets standards generated from an interaction of their personalities and their professional training. The responsibility to be a good physician is deeply rooted in professionalism, arising from the idealism of the beginning student, and nurtured and reinforced by medical faculty and practicing physicians who served as role models during the years of training. The standards for performance that result from this process are fundamentally similar, but they may also differ. In some areas of practice, individual physicians may express standards that are far higher than their colleagues', because in these areas they desire to excel, to lead their field. In others, what is commonly held as best for the patient is accepted and established as a goal for clinical performance. Physicians are also trained and socialized to value the knowledge and skills which lie at the heart of their clinical performance. Having an adequate body of knowledge and skill becomes a preordinate standard, because it is seen as so instrumental to performing well. Physicians often see knowledge and skill as predictive of clinical effectiveness.

Ways of practicing which are best today may not be best tomorrow. A plethora of books and articles describing the ways practices should be changed to provide patients with better care repeatedly make physicians feel that they must change in order to meet their own standards of performance. In tandem, the presence of new and better ways and the discrediting of previously acceptable ways of practicing medicine generate an imperative for "keeping up to date." This personal interpretation of the socially sanctioned standards of performance is fundamental to self-evaluation. It is this tension between the desire to do what is "one's best," and the changing intrepretations of what is "best," that drives the 184 changes described in this chapter.

Nearly all the physicians interviewed for this study provided changes related to their clinical practices. While many of these changes were driven by pressures from the social and clinical environment, or from personal needs and desires of the physician, the largest single group of changes was driven primarily by the desire for a sense of competence or excellence. Moreover, from an overview of the changes described in all of these chapters, one suspects that this motivation pervades all of the changes to some extent, even when the drive for competence was not the primary force for change. The rationale behind analyzing these changes as a group is that the desire to do "one's best" was described by these physicians as the primary cause for making changes. In some cases, the wish to do "one's best" singularly led to a change. In others, some external factor was necessary to release the energy to change, energy that came either from increasingly unacceptable patient outcomes or an innovation which promised to be more effective.

FACTORS PRODUCING CHANGE

By itself, the desire to excel led the physician to make 17.4 percent (32 of 184) of the changes in this chapter. Examples of changes resulting from these purely internal, personal expectations came from physicians of all ages and specialties. For example, an orthopedic surgeon, early in his career, "wanted to excel in a particular area" of his specialty and so focused his attention on practice and research in sports medicine and spinal surgery. A radiologist, relatively late in his career, worked hard to gain competence in the use of ultrasound equipment, so that he might "remain at the head of his specialty." A young family physician, who had started to practice recently, sought opportunities to gain skill and confidence in insertion of intrauterine devices (IUD's) because she felt that she, as a family physician, should be able to do this contraceptive procedure in her own office to "provide complete care." These examples illustrate how striving to meet personal standards of what ought to be done can cause physicians to seek new ways to improve.

In other cases, the drive to do "one's best" was triggered either by the presence of an innovation that allowed for improved care or by a growing dissatisfaction with the results of currently used methods of providing care. The largest single category of competency-based changes (100 of 184, 54.3 percent) resulted from a combination of the personal drive to do one's best and the presence of an innovation allowing for improved care. New information, procedures, drugs, technologies, and equipment all contributed to these changes. Another 28.3 percent (52 of 184) of the changes were attributed to the physicians' growing dissatisfaction with current procedures and treatments in tandem with the desire to perform better. Most commonly, the stage was set for change when physicians had experienced difficulties in the care of a number of patients with the same kinds of problems. For example, after receiving four positive Pap smear reports regarding patients who had negative smears shortly before, one physician shortened the interval between re-examinations. Another physician's dissatisfaction with his results in management of angina patients set the stage for the adoption of calcium channel blockers when he heard about them in a lecture. Yet another felt embarrassed by his inadequacy in taking sexual histories, so when the need to do so increased because of changes in his patient load, he sought more information and skill in this area.

Therefore, the drive for competent performance in patient care is manifest in three ways:

1. Physicians make some changes because it is part of living up to their high personal standards for professional behavior.
2. Physicians may be open to change and do so as soon as there is some innovation, some new or better way of practicing.
3. Physicians sometimes become dissatisfied with current procedures or outcomes because these do not match with what they think is "best," so they look for a more acceptable alternative.

It is valuable to observe the difference in the nature of these three pressures to change. In the case of the first, changing because the physician wishes to remain at the leading edge of his or her field implied an ongoing drive to constantly upgrade knowledge and skills in performance—a kind of perpetual energy. In the second case, initiation of change indicated an ongoing receptivity to change that is dependent upon the presence of a relevant innovation. The third is driven by the need to develop practices with more desirable outcomes; in effect, change is stimulated by a specific problem. In the first situation change is constantly sought; in the second, a continuing openness to change is present; and in the third, change is episodic, and dependent upon how practices and especially patient outcomes conflict with personal and professional standards. But in all, no change would occur without the basic, intrinsic desire to be a competent physician.

TYPES OF CHANGES

Most of the forces for change described in this study brought about a range of accommodations, adjustments, redirections, and perspective transformations rather than consistently leading to only one or two of these types of changes. However, this was not the case when change was driven by the desire for competence. These changes were adjustments in the physicians' practices rather than accommodations, redirections, or perspective transformations. This overwhelming tendency to make smaller, more controlled changes is reasonable, given the slow and careful way advances are made in clinical science and clinical practice. The dramatic breakthroughs that would compel physicians to make major changes in their approaches to medicine are rare. Adjusting one's practice requires not only feeling the pressure to change, but also thinking about what is to be changed, and adapting, rather than adopting or accommodating, a different way. Adjustment-type changes would seem to be the likely outcome of the change process in these cases because, by definition, these changes are thoughtful but cautious attempts to bring about a better fit between "what is" and "what ought to be," rather than passively accepting a way of practicing, or actively restructuring life or practice.

WHAT CHANGED?

Although prescribing habits and procedures were the most common areas to be altered, there was a surprisingly wide assortment of changes across the spectrum of clinical care. There were changes in history-taking and physical examinations, and in ordering of laboratory and radiological investigations. Changes also occurred in how the doctors organized their practices, how they taught students, and how they thought and felt about their profession. One family physician responded to recent information in the literature regarding lifestyle and risk factors by incorporating questions on smoking and exercise into his routine histories. Another changed the way he examined male genitalia after attending a conference on physical examination. A surprising number of physicians reported changes related to preventive measures. One family physician, in mid-career, recognized the importance of organizing his patient charts in such a way that they provided him "keys" for necessary periodic care—reminders for timely screening procedures and other data that helped him act in a positive way in the area of health promotion, regardless of the patient's presenting complaint at any specific visit.

In managing patient problems, the most common change was in prescribing practices (57 of 184 changes reported in this chapter). Most of those (37 of 57) came about because the physician became aware of a new drug or new information about an old drug, largely from literature. The remaining changes related to prescribing were described as resulting from physician dissatisfaction with results of previous therapy, such as side effects or inadequate results.

LEARNING

Of all the changes discovered in this study, those driven by the desire for competence were more likely than all others to involve learning. In ninety-two percent of the cases where change was driven by the desire for competence, learning was described as a means for change. The remainder of the cases presumably required no new knowledge or skills. This is in marked contrast to changes caused by all other forces, where approximately seventy-one percent (553 of 775) of the changes were associated with recent learning.

New learning was described most often as directed toward solving a problem (60 percent of cases), the remainder being for the purpose of gaining a better conceptual understanding (40 percent). The proportion of problem-oriented learning was slightly greater when the motivation for change was a difficulty managing patients (76 percent), or when the change in practice behavior involved implementing a new procedure (77 percent). Similarly, physicians demonstrated a marked preference (74 percent) for learning that incorporated actual involvement, interaction, or experience, in making changes when the element of practice being changed was a procedure, compared with fifty-three percent of all the changes in the project. The alternative type of learning, that emphasized deliberation rather than experience, was predominant in only twenty-six percent of procedural changes, but forty-seven percent of all changes.

The preference for formal resources over informal ones was slightly greater in competence-related changes (80 percent) than in the total project data (66 percent). The proportion was higher (84 percent) when the changes were made as a result of the awareness of innovation, and higher yet (88.5 percent) when the element of practice changed was investigation prior to diagnosis. Conversely, informal resources played a proportionally larger role when new procedures were being learned.

While most changes were associated with a relatively well-defined, discrete learning strategy, a subset of twenty changes were described in sufficient detail to allow us to recognize the different ways that learning was used in three different phases of change. The case below illustrates three separate phases observed in the learning associated with those twenty changes.

Two years ago I began to use laser surgery to remove skin lesions. I had seen patients with tattoos and port wine lesions before that time, but I was frustrated because I had no treatment for them. In the previous two or three years, I read numerous articles in the *Archives of Dermatology* and other journals, describing how laser surgery could be used to remove tattoos and a host of other skin lesions, and I was impressed by the effectiveness and safety of the procedure. At a local dermatology meeting, I discussed the possibility of obtaining a laser therapy unit with six of my colleagues, and then later, with our hospital administration. We convinced the hospital that investing in a laser therapy unit would be economically and medically beneficial. Before buying the equipment, however, I arranged for an out-of-state dermatologist friend to conduct a four-hour meeting on the technique of using laser therapy for skin lesions. Sales representatives from three different instrument companies brought their equipment to the hospital and conducted demonstrations. After purchasing the unit of our choice, I was ready to do laser surgery. Once we had the equipment, I arranged for another dermatologist friend, a recognized authority in laser surgery, to help me and my colleagues develop our skills for this new procedure. He spent a full week at our hospital, giving a course for the dermatologists. Six of us brought patients to the hospital and did laser surgery under his supervision. During that week I did six of my own cases and observed colleagues doing 24 other cases. After this "hands-on" experience, I felt competent to perform laser surgery without further supervision. I felt I still had not learned enough yet. A short time later, I participated in a continuing medical education conference on dermatology, where laser therapy was discussed. From that meeting, I learned about other conditions that could be treated with the laser.

This 35-year-old dermatologist illustrates how different types of learning may be employed in making a change in practice. He worked through three distinct phases of learning in order to adopt this new surgical procedure. These phases were: (1) preparing to change, (2) making the change, and (3) solidifying the change. Before committing himself to laser surgery, he prepared to change by reading journal articles, attending a CME meeting, discussing this innovation with six of his colleagues, and meeting with hospital administrators. Having decided to adopt the procedure and buy the equipment, he pursued other learning activities to help him actually make this change. He met with equipment representatives and arranged for two different laser surgery experts to share their knowledge with him and his colleagues at the hospital. Then, having begun to use the procedure without supervision, he solidified this change by learning additional uses for laser therapy at a dermatology conference.

A number of physicians in this chapter went through similar phases in their learning. They first engaged in a variety of learning activities that eventually *prepared them to change* some aspects of their professional or personal lives. These activities led to a decision: Whether to adopt a new diagnostic procedure, prescribe a new drug, use a new surgical technique, or not. Once they had decided to *make the change,* a different phase of learning began. Learning activities in this second phase were designed to increase their knowledge of the new drug or develop their skills in using the new procedure. Confident to proceed on their own, a third phase began. While prescribing the new drug or using the new procedure, they continued to learn in ways that *solidified the change* that had been made. This section concentrates on the twenty physicians who clearly proceeded through all three phases of learning: Preparing to change, making the

Table 6.1
Learning Resources Used During "Preparing to Change" Phase

Learning Resource	Number of Physicians N = 20
Continuing Medical Education Programs	15
Journal Reading	12
Interaction with Other Physicians	12
Use of Other Instructional Materials	6
Interaction with Non-Physicians	5

change, and solidifying the change. These cases were selected for a closer look, because these physicians described their learning activities with considerably more detail than the other physicians examined in this chapter.

PREPARING TO CHANGE

Physicians driven to change by a desire to remain professionally competent used a variety of learning activities to prepare themselves to change. They learned from various CME programs, from reading journals, from using other instructional materials, from other physicians, and from non-physicians. Table 6.1 shows how each of these learning resources was used by our subset of twenty physicians during the preparing-to-change phase.

Participation in a formally organized CME activity was the most frequent way these physicians prepared to change. Fifteen of the twenty physicians had participated in at least one CME activity during this initial phase. Some participated in several different types of CME. Practically every variety of CME was reported, from weekly grand rounds to intensive, skill development courses. As noted above, the dermatologist found a small, local dermatologists' meeting a good place to discuss with colleagues the possibility of doing laser surgery. A psychiatrist, who is now using a new antidepressant drug, gained information about it during the weekly grand rounds sponsored by a university psychiatry department. A radiologist first heard about ultrasound technology as a resident, during a joint meeting between his hospital and a nearby university hospital.

Meetings sponsored by professional associations were also important. For example, a pathologist, who changed her routine in examining bladder specimens for carcinoma following total cystectomy of the urinary bladder, first considered this change after hearing it discussed at a state pathology meeting. A plastic

Table 6.2
Learning Resources Used During "Making the Change" Phase

Learning Resource	Number of Physicians N = 20
Interaction with Other Physicians	10
Continuing Medical Education Program	6
Use of Other Instructional Materials	4
Journal Reading	3
Interaction with Non-Physicians	2

surgeon, now doing liposuction, heard helpful talks on the topic at a meeting of the American Society of Plastic and Reconstructive Surgery. Courses where specific diagnostic procedures or treatments were presented, or reviewed, were useful for some physicians. A family practitioner, who had begun to use the non-stress test in prenatal care to diagnose fetal maturity and uterine readiness, began to think about changing practices in obstetrics while participating in an OB/GYN refresher course at his local university. Farther from home, an ophthalmologist, who now inserts intraocular lenses, first began to prepare himself to do this procedure during a course he took in London, England. This course consisted of one-on-one teaching in the operating room.

During the preparation phase, reasons for participating in CME differed. Some physicians attended meetings to gain specific information. An orthopedic surgeon, who has begun doing acromioplasty for relief of tendon impingement beneath the acromion, went to an academy meeting to learn more about this new surgical procedure. A cardiologist, considering adoption of the two-dimensional echo technique, went to a four-day symposium devoted to this procedure, because it was run by the best leaders on echo technique in the country. He came back, in his word, "converted." Other physicians, however, did not have a preconceived learning agenda. The previously mentioned pathologist heard a speaker at a state meeting present findings for tumors of the genito-urinary tract. The speaker noted that sectioning the entire urethral specimen following cystectomy sometimes led to finding residual malignancy. This information was new to her, and she began to consider changing her examination procedures.

All of these examples involved participation in just one CME meeting. The ophthalmologist now doing lens insertions, however, is an example of someone for whom many meetings were a significant part of the preparation phase. His study of implantation surgery coincided with what he described as a "general international debate on the pros and cons of implantation surgery which went on for several years." As a result, he was "bombarded" with information on the topic at every meeting he attended.

Twelve of the twenty physicians described becoming aware of some new diagnostic procedure or treatment through reading. The radiologist now using ultrasound, for example, began subscribing to the *Journal of Ultrasound*. For two years he and his partner read this journal faithfully, and discussed the possibility of getting their own machine.

Twelve physicians, eight of whom relied on peers or colleagues, learned from other physicians. Four of these eight learned from their partners, or members of their clinic groups. One partner had just joined a group of anesthesiologists. He had trained at a hospital where nasal tubes were inserted in cases of epiglottitis. Since a considerable amount of discussion took place every day in this group of anesthesiologists, he soon began to share what he had learned in his residency. These discussions led to other learning activities for the anesthesiologist who eventually adopted this procedure. Another partner helped an orthopedic surgeon learn to do acromioplasty. After an orthopedic academy meeting about the new shoulder operation, he shared the information on returning to the clinic. His other partner then proceeded to learn more about the procedure.

Other examples included learning from out-of-town colleagues. A gastroen-terologist visiting a former schoolmate, and residency colleague, saw him insert a gastrotomy feeding tube. And as proof that learning is not confined to the classroom, office, or study, another orthopedic surgeon discussed cementless joints with a colleague while mountain climbing.

Half of those who learned from other physicians during this phase tapped the knowledge of recognized experts in a particular area. Two of these experts were consultants to whom a physician had referred patients. After the family practi-tioner now using the non-stress test in prenatal care had attended the refresher course, he noted that several consultants were ordering these tests. Their formal consultation letters were an important part of his subsequent decision to order them himself.

In additional to journals, six physicians used a variety of other instructional materials. Four physicians reviewed textbooks on a particular topic, typically in conjunction with other forms of learning. Two physicians viewed videotapes which had been produced to illustrate specific procedures. One physician used pharmaceutical advertising to add to his knowledge of a particular drug.

People other than physicians were learning resources for five physicians as they prepared to change. Two physicians reported that pharmaceutical represen-tatives helped them consider whether to use a new drug. The above-mentioned dermatologist noted that an equipment representative played a role when he was adopting laser surgery. The radiologist now using ultrasound stated that an itinerant ultrasonographer, who came to his clinic on a regular basis, taught him about the new technology. A faculty member in pediatrics, who developed a new approach to teaching medical students, benefited from an educator who critiqued his ideas in the formative stages.

Preparing to Change Summary

This first phase affirms the value of the traditional methods of learning in medicine. The three most frequently reported learning resources were CME programs, journals, and informal interaction with other physicians. Formal programs were the most frequently used. Although traditional resources were the most important, five of the twenty physicians indicated they learned from interaction with people other than physicians. The preparation phase can be characterized as "taking it all in." Physicians absorbed information from a variety of resources. On average, each of the twenty physicians used two to three different types of learning resources. Some used the same resource, CME programs for example, several different times.

Learning activities during the first phase were often reported in great detail. Several physicians described a litany of learning activities spanning a period as long as five years. On the other hand, the preparing-to-change period was sometimes quite short, and could involve a single learning activity.

MAKING THE CHANGE

At a certain point, a physician felt sufficiently prepared to change. He or she had learned enough about a new drug or surgical procedure, for example, and was ready to begin a second learning phase. In *making the change,* learning became more focused as the physician developed specific skills or gained new information. For example, the dermatologist, after the decision was made to buy the laser equipment, began to prepare himself to do the laser surgery on his own. He arranged for two laser experts to come to the hospital to teach him and his colleagues more about the procedure. He also discussed equipment with three sales representatives.

As with the previous phase, the twenty physicians used a variety of learning activities while making the change. Unlike the previous phase, they used fewer learning resources. Table 6.2 shows how many physicians used each of these types of learning activities and resources during the second phase.

As in the preparation phase, peers were a more frequent learning resource than experts during the making-the-change phase. For example, the anesthesiologist, who had begun to insert nasal tubes in cases of epiglottitis, developed his skills while working with other colleagues. During a three-month period, he tried the technique for himself three different times in the hospital setting. He inserted the first one while working with an ear, nose, and throat specialist, and the last two in collaboration with another anesthesiologist. After these three insertions, he felt much more comfortable with the procedure and was able to proceed more on his own. Six of the ten physicians who reported learning from other physicians described peer interactions as a means for learning. The other four physicians made use of recognized experts, including local faculty members and national leaders. The family practitioner continued to utilize her residency instructor as she learned to insert IUD's on her own. The orthopedist, on the other hand, decided to try cementless joints. He contacted an expert he had met at a national orthopedic meeting and arranged to spend twenty-four hours with him at his hospital. During this time, he scrubbed in surgery, witnessed one hip surgery, and did one hip surgery under the expert's supervision. This one-on-one experience was extremely valuable for him. It was a real test of learning how to solve problems when they occurred.

Although used less extensively than in the preparation phase, formal CME programs were an important resource. Six physicians acknowledged the role CME played, four citing local programs, while two traveled to gather the information. For example, while developing his skills to insert intraocular lenses, the ophthalmologist found a local course sponsored jointly by a regional ophthalmology association and the university to be very helpful. It was a "hands-on" course that both demonstrated the techniques and then allowed practicing two different ways to implant lenses on eye models. The ultrasonic radiologist heard of an excellent course given by a highly regarded pioneer in the field. Before attending the course, he reviewed his ultrasound journals to make the most of the two weeks he would spend with the expert. He also read a book on imaging, and took several others on the subject to study in the evenings.

Finally, a family practitioner, who began to prescribe calcium antagonists, found three different CME activities useful. During the time he was making the change, he attended five local sessions describing the use of calcium antagonists. These sessions included dinner meetings sponsored by drug companies, local hospital rounds, and other lecture presentations held in his community. He then attended two refresher courses and a one-day program at the local medical school. In marked contrast to the first phase, journal reading was much less frequent. Only three physicians acknowledged the use of journals. One physician who did find journal articles useful was the orthopedic surgeon now performing acromioplasty. Having decided to do this type of shoulder surgery, he studied the journal *Clinical Orthopedics* for at least ten hours before attempting his first case.

Videotapes were also used in this phase, as mentioned by two of the four physicians who used instructional material. Only two physicians used people who were non-physicians as learning resources.

Making the Change Summary

Traditional learning resources were important during this second phase of learning, but they were used less frequently. Informal interaction with other physicians replaced CME programs as the most used resource, and was only

Table 6.3
Learning Resources Used During "Solidifying the Change" Phase

Learning Resource	Number of Physicians N = 20
Interaction with Other Physicians	11
Continuing Medical Education	8
Journal Reading	8
Teaching	5
Use of Other Instructional Materials	4
Interaction with Non-Physicians	3

slightly less frequent than in the first phase. CME and journal reading, however, were significantly less important. *Making the change* can be characterized as "taking the plunge." Learning was more active than in the first phase, as physicians experimented and tested their newly acquired skills or information. Fewer types of learning resources were used, on average just over one per physician. In this phase, then, physicians indicated a more intensive use of fewer resources.

SOLIDIFYING THE CHANGE

Even after physicians have made a change, their needs for learning continue. They may feel competent to perform a certain procedure or prescribe a new drug, but a new procedure or drug prescription must become a habit. This habit is developed through continuing practice with the procedure or drug prescription, along with evaluation of the results. At times, a procedure needs to be modified, or additional uses of a new drug are realized. During this phase of learning, the physicians solidify the changes that have been made, making them established parts of their practices.

As in previous phases, the twenty physicians participated in a variety of learning activities that helped them solidify the changes they had made. The dermatologist felt competent to perform laser surgery without further supervision. Yet, he did not stop learning about it. He attended a conference where laser surgery was discussed, learning of other conditions that could be treated with the laser. Table 6.3 indicates the learning resources used, and how many physicians used them.As the table indicates, eleven physicians learned from other physicians during this third phase, similar to the first and second phases. Unlike the other phases, a greater proportion of physicians relied on their peers or colleagues as learning resources, than relied on experts or consultants. In this phase, ten of the eleven physicians (91 percent) learned from their colleagues, compared to eight of twelve (67 percent) in the first phase and six of ten (60 percent) in the second phase.

Partners were the most obvious, and perhaps the most readily available, learning resources. Three physicians had partners who helped them solidify a change they had implemented. The orthopedic surgeon, now doing acromioplasty, had the benefit of three partners. After he began doing this shoulder operation, his partners began doing similar surgeries. The four physicians discussed their results frequently. The radiologist, now doing ultrasound imaging, continued to learn from his partner as they reviewed all of their cases together. The family practitioner, now making increased use of the nonstress test, found ongoing discussion with other family practitioners in his group to be helpful in solidifying this change.

Others learned from colleagues who were not their practice partners. The pediatrics faculty member found ongoing discussions with other faculty members helpful, as he solidified the changes he had made in teaching medical students. The orthopedic surgeon performing cementless total joint replacements found discussions with a colleague at the local medical school helpful, as he spent time in the laboratory trying different techniques. The anesthesiologist, who now inserts nasal tubes in cases of epiglottitis, completed six more tube insertions and learned from ear, nose, and throat specialists, as well as anesthesiologists who worked with him on the insertions.

Only two physicians learned from experts or consultants during this phase. One, the family physician, learned from both peers and experts. She learned more about IUDs from discussions with other family physicians and with gynecologists to whom she referred difficult cases.

As in the previous two phases, formally-organized CME activities continued to be an important learning resource, but local CME activities played a larger role during this phase. For at least four of the eight physicians who found CME helpful, local or state meetings were an important learning resource. The family practitioner, inserting IUDs, found her hospital's obstetrical rounds to be an excellent forum to discuss issues related to IUDs and other OB/GYN topics. After declining in importance as a learning resource in the second phase, journals were used more frequently for solidifying change. Eight of the twenty physicians cited journal reading as helpful.

Noteworthy for the solidification phase is the use of teaching as an additional learning resource. After a physician has made a change, opportunities occur to teach others about a new treatment or procedure. While preparing to teach, and during the teaching, the physician is learning more about the change he or she has made. As the saying goes, "The best way to learn something is to teach it."

In solidifying change, five of the twenty physicians engaged in some kind of teaching activity. The dermatologist developed handouts about laser surgery and taught his patients and his nurses about it. Four other physicians taught colleagues about the changes they had made. The gastroenterologist, who inserts gastrotomy feeding tubes, taught his partner to perform the procedure. Another gastroenterologist, who learned the Endoscopic Retrograde Cholangiopan creatography (ERCP) procedure, taught other physicians how to do it. The psychiatrist, now using a new antidepressant drug, is the only psychiatrist working in the student health unit, where other physicians meet each other in the corridor or at lunch and talk about patient problems. In this setting, he is a teacher of these colleagues, particularly about the new drug and the psychopharmacology of other psychotropic medication. The cardiologist who adopted the two-dimensional echocardiographic technique, now teaches the reading of echoes at CME conferences. These examples all show the role teaching plays in learning to solidify change.

Four of the twenty physicians learned from other instructional materials. These materials included books describing specific procedures, a monthly medical letter, monthly university pharmacy bulletins, reprints from pharmaceutical representatives, as well as video tapes demonstrating a particular technique.

Solidifying the Change Summary

Traditional learning resources continued to be important in the third phase. Informal interaction with other physicians retained its most-favored frequency status and was used about as often as in the previous two phases. CME and journal reading were used frequently, although not as often as in the first phase. Local resources were used more often than in the previous two phases. Physicians sought interaction with physicians who practiced in their clinics or communities. Although they might have learned new skills from an acknowledged international expert, they worked with their colleagues back home to integrate these skills into their practices. They also found local CME meetings an important place for discussing approaches to patient problems.

The solidifying-the-change phase can be characterized as "reaching out." Physicians "reached out" to learn from their local colleagues and CME meetings. More significantly, they "reached out" through teaching opportunities. Teaching both solidified their learning and furthered the dissemination of change in the local community.

CONCLUSIONS: DISCUSSION AND IMPLICATIONS

We have seen that change is pervasive in medical practice. Experienced clinicians respond to a variety of pressures by seeking information from numerous sources before, during, and after implementing a change. Following are conclusions regarding change as a function of the desire for competence and excellence.

The desire of physicians for competence was manifest in three forms: A desire to excell or be the "best" in one's field, an openness to change with innovation, and a willingness to react to problems encountered in clinical practice.

The intrinsic need to provide patients with the very best care possible is a powerful motivation for change in clinical practice. The three orientations to change were clearly revealed in the interviews, but it was unclear whether the orientation to change was general or situation-specific. It was clear that, in some physicians in some situations, the motivation to change was activated only when a specific problem was encountered. This problem-specific orientation to change was a relatively common phenomenon, occurring sometimes in quick response to a particular experience, but also, in some cases, not until several patients exhibited the same problem. Physicians are expected to change when evidence indicates unsatisfactory clinical outcomes, but the interviews did not reveal the extent to which some physicians may use this approach predominantly or even exclusively.

An openness to change, coupled with the awareness of a desirable innovation, provided the largest group of changes driven by the desire for competence. The distinction here was that the trigger was an opportunity to change as the result of something external to the physician, as contrasted with a willingness to change as a result of a problem. Physicians making changes as a result of this approach showed evidence of an ongoing internalized desire to be up-to-date, a personal standard adopted during the process of "professionalization."

The third orientation to change was characterized by an active, affirmative desire for change, in an ongoing search for excellence. In contrast to the other two types, this searching for excellence appeared to be personal, requiring neither a problem nor the awareness of an innovation in the environment. These physicians actively sought ways to be better, to be on the "cutting edge" of change. This was, however, the most infrequent orientation to change. Although it may appear highly desirable for physicians to approach change in this way, there also may be negative consequences unless it is coupled with a thorough understanding of when the "new way" is a "better way." Again, it was unclear whether those physicians who described this orientation operate in this mode most of the time, or whether they use it in certain areas or specific situations in their practices. For example, it may be that a particular family physician would *seek* changes in sports medicine and be *open* to incorporating new beta-blockers in the management of angina, yet wait until *problems* confront him or her in patients with rheumatoid arthritis. It may be that the optimal situation occurs when a physician is able to utilize all three approaches to change depending upon a given situation.

Physicians making changes driven by the desire for competence overwhelmingly "adjust" elements of practice, including a broad range of clinical activities from history-taking to surgical procedures. Medical practice evolves step by step. A hesitancy to react to every new idea or bit of information is part of a basic conservative approach to the practice of medicine that is taught and modeled in the training years of physicians. Probably, this approach preserves the mandate to "do no harm." As this incremental approach serves to protect patients, it also may retard appropriate changes. Occasionally, significant reorientations in thinking and new directions in practices are needed. An example of this is in the area of geriatrics. Here, physicians must learn that the same illness cannot be treated identically in young and old patients. There is a need to approach the elderly patient in a completely different way, focusing on assisting him or her to cope with changes of aging, with a goal of maximizing function rather than curing disease. This will require some primary care physicians to transform their approaches to the whole patient, and some consultants may need to redirect components of their practices by gaining new skills and taking on responsibility for larger numbers of ill elderly. The wide variety of practice elements that changed was surprising. Finding changes in history-taking, record keeping, preventive aspects of healthcare, and the teaching of students, reassures us that physicians have not focused too much on traditional "curative" aspects of practice—prescription drugs and procedures.

When physicians made changes driven by the desire for competence, they engaged in activities to learn something new in the overwhelming majority (92 percent) of cases. The differences between the proportions of changes dependent upon learning in this chapter and those in other chapters were dramatic. Physicians are trained to consider learning an essential part of the evolution of their practices and an elaborate system of rounds, refresher courses, professional association meetings, journals, audio-visual instructional materials, and texts exists to provide learning opportunities. Physicians know how to select and use resources and there is a general expectation that they will do so.

In some circumstances, learning was a more complex, three-phase process with a different mix of learning activities in each. Three phases were clearly seen in many changes described in the interviews: Learning directed toward "preparing to change," "making the change," and "solidifying the change." It is likely that many other of the learning projects included all three phases, but the information was not offered by the physicians and the interviews did not seek details to elaborate these phases. One major difference among these phases of learning was the types of learning resources used. "Preparing to change" was typified by use of many different resources. Formally organized CME programs were the most commonly used resource, followed closely by journals and other physicians (colleagues in an informal situation). However, when physicians were "making the change," colleagues were by far the most frequently used resource, with journals and formal programs dropping substantially. After the change had been made, "solidifying change" involved colleagues foremost, with journals and formally organized programs rising again, but not to the level of importance seen in "preparing to change."

Other physicians in informal settings, both peers and consultants, were very important learning resources in all three phases. Formally organized CME programs were critical in preparing physicians for change. They provided new information or, in some cases, confirmation of the need to change. Although they were less frequent when the physician was making the change, they helped later when he or she was confirming the appropriateness of the move. Similarly, journals were very important in the preparation phase but of little use in the process of changing. Like CME programs, they were somewhat more helpful when a physician was solidifying change.

The three phases of learning help us better understand how CME relates to the process of change. We often wonder about the value of programs, and whether they have an effect on the physicians who participate. The teachers and those who fund these programs would like to show that specific CME programs have an impact on the practice of medicine. For example, a study conducted by Sibley et al. (1982) investigated the impact of continuing education packages on the overall quality of care, with discouraging results.

The radiologist who began to use ultrasound is an excellent example of someone who was prepared to make a change. After a two-week ultrasound course, he began using this procedure in his practice. Yet, before the course, he and his partner had read extensively about this area, and had decided to buy the necessary equipment.

Physicians attend CME programs at different phases in the change process. Some, as a direct result of participating in a CME program, go back home and make changes in some aspect of their practices right away. These physicians readily show the effect CME programs have on the delivery of healthcare. Our interviews suggest, however, that these physicians may already be planning this change before they come to the program. They may be in the second phase of learning—"making the change"—and are seeking specific skills or information to help them "get over the hump." They get what they need and go home to use it.

Not all physicians who attend CME programs are at the same stage of readiness to change; many still are "preparing to change." They are considering a possible change and use a CME meeting as one type of learning resource. Because the majority of CME participants may be in the initial learning phase, an experiment that measures behavior change immediately after this course will find no major change. Yet, our interviews asserted that such a program can make an important contribution to changing. Other physicians who participate in CME programs have already made changes. They come to programs to solidify their gains. These physicians will also show no major changes in any experimental evaluation. Instead, they find that the program helped to confirm or reinforce the value of what they are already doing. In essence, there is no opportunity to change.

RECOMMENDATIONS

The three approaches to change, willingness to change in response to problems, openness to change in response to innovation, and a desire to excel, need more research to further clarify their natures. Do individual physicians operate in all three modes at different times and in different situations, or do they change predominantly with one approach or another? Is there a relationship between approach to change and personality type, specialty, or "learning style"? And perhaps, most importantly, is there a relationship between orientation to change and the learning resources used to prepare for, make, and solidify that change? Can physicians be taught to vary their orientations to change in different situations?

CME program providers need to recognize that physicians attend their courses for varied reasons. Some will be there to seek information to solve specific patient problems. Is it necessary to offer problem-solving formats to assist them in incorporating the new knowledge or skill, or are their specific patient problems an adequate framework? Will they learn efficiently from didactic lectures? Other physicians may be present with no specific patient problems but simply because their personal standards of keeping up to date require them to acquire new information to incorporate when the opportunity presents itself.

Regarding the types of changes made in physicians' practices, research is needed to clarify the exact nature of the changes we have labelled as "adjustments." In this broad category, we have lumped together changing from one drug to another of the same class, and new surgical procedures. There is obviously a considerable difference in these changes, and, presumably, the learning required to make them, and the facilitating and inhibiting factors will be different. How can physicians be encouraged to make the broader changes, redirection or transformations, when needed? CME program providers in Geriatrics/Gerontology, for example, would benefit from the answers to this question.

Because physicians are engaged in new learning with nearly every change driven by their desire for competence, anyone wishing to change physician behavior in an area of clinical competence should build in an opportunity for learning, if he or she wishes to succeed. Individuals in hospital management positions who wish to improve some element of care in their institutions will be unlikely to succeed by edict alone. Licensing bodies attempting to deal with physicians whose competence has slipped need to plan for education in a most careful manner.

Physicians themselves must also recognize the strong relationship between new learning and change and, consequently, maintain a system for easy and accurate access to information. For example, they should be able to store and retrieve important articles or notes from courses, and use library resources in their own institutions, or via one of the online computer systems available to them.

The variable mix of learning resources in the three phases of learning leads us to our final set of recommendations. The most important resource, when all three phases are considered, was one's colleagues or peers. Consequently, we must do further research to clarify how their roles in the process can be facilitated. Earlier research (Hiss, et al. 1979) on "educational influentials," that is, respected colleagues in the medical community, focused on using community doctors to disseminate new information to other physicians, with the expectations that innovation would thus be introduced and adopted. Our interviews suggest that the efforts might have been more efficient if physicians who were in the process of making a change were assisted by these "educational influentials." Presumably, we can train "educational influentials" in these techniques, and make them more effective. One would also presume that learning together would help peers help each other through the second and third phases, and thus, we would recommend that more local programming be oriented toward a community of physicians rather than, for example, specialty subsets. When primary care physicians and their consultant colleagues learn together, it is likely that change will be facilitated. CME program providers must recognize that physicians in all three phases of learning may be present in their audiences, and that a significant number may be preparing to change, or consolidating changes already made. Research is needed to clarify what implications this has for the content of programs and their organization. Certainly, the role of peers in the process should be acknowledged by teachers in these programs.

CME researchers should reconsider their attempts to evaluate the impact of one educational intervention. We must recognize the complex, multifaceted nature of physician behavior change in clinical matters and design evaluation protocols that more accurately reflect the roles of CME programs in all three phases of change.

REFERENCES

Hiss, R. G., et al. 1979. Development and evaluation of a community-based pulmonary education system. *Proceedings of the 18th Annual Conference on Research in Medical Education,* Washington, D.C., November 1979:264–269.

Sibley, J. C., et al. 1982. A randomized trial of continuing medical education. *New England Journal of Medicine* 306:511–515.

7

The Clinical Environment

David Davis

I work out twice a week in a racquet club, and many of the people I play squash with have become my patients. Their commonest complaint, as you might imagine, is tennis elbow, for which I used to prescribe ice or heat, ultrasound and anti-inflammatory medication. This wasn't always successful: The treatment was slow and often ineffective, and my patients, politely enough, would demand "the cortisone injection." I was reluctant at first, but I picked up an orthopedics text one day in the hospital library and reviewed the anatomy of elbows, and then saw a course called "Orthopedics Workshop 1986" at a nearby medical school. I attended the program and took the workshops on shoulder and elbow injections (with mannequins and 2 actual patients in each). Feeling more comfortable now with the procedure, I've done several in my office. I've even begun to think about opening an evening clinic in sports medicine, right at the racquet club.

Recently, I moved my practice from a small house in the suburbs to a larger and more modern office downtown, closer to the hospital where I do most of my referral work. My patients were changing. Fifteen years ago, I started practice in the "growth area" of this community, the suburbs. Over the last ten years, however, I noticed that some of my "empty nest" patients were moving away, often into the core of the city. On top of that, many other new internists and subspecialists had come to the suburbs, competing for new patients. And it was getting harder to get to the downtown hospital where I practice, because of traffic. So, I talked to a real estate agent, and consulted with two members in my call group. We talked through a possible move and did some financial planning with a real estate agent and an accountant. Finally, we decided to move into a relatively new office building, which contained x-ray facilities and a laboratory (a convenience which my old building didn't have). I feel very good about this change. I can get to the hospital in half the time, order laboratory tests and x-rays done in the same building (in fact, I like reading x-rays myself), and my patients seem much happier as well. I have also noticed a shift in my patient load—more young unmarried patients and geriatric cases, both of which have prompted some learning on my part.

One relatively common stereotype of the physician portrays him or her as self-contained and independent, and packed with knowledge and skill gained in undergraduate and graduate training. This package is modified to some extent as clinical experience is acquired and as inner-directed motivation leads to accomplishment. From this viewpoint, the doctor applies a universal set of medical standards to the circumstances he or she encounters—the doctor being little influenced by those circumstances.

That view is naive. The milieu in which a doctor practices comprises several forces for change. Among these are pressures from staff or patients, economic or administrative issues affecting the purchase or use of equipment and facilities, competition from colleagues, and learning opportunities. We have chosen the term *clinical environment* to characterize this set of forces for change, but we equally well might have chosen the term *workplace*. The clinical environment has two distinct but related dimensions: (1) patients (consumers) and (2) the delivery system, which includes other providers of healthcare, the equipment and materials that are used for delivery of patient care, and the information which undergirds care.

Without appropriate support facilities or structures, even the best-intentioned or most educated physician will fail to employ adequate patient care practices. For example, chlamydia is thought to be responsible for up to forty percent of gynecologic infections and subsequent infertility (Sweet 1988). Although this fact may be well-known, few physicians giving primary care perform the appropriate tests because, they report, many laboratories and offices lack proper culture media or means to transport and store them at optimum temperatures.

The working environment powerfully constrains the behavior of physicians. Studies of the effects of formal CME have indicated that courses ''work,'' that is, produce changes in knowledge or performance, only when they are attuned to needs arising from the clinical environment (Davis et al. 1984). Change occurring in the context of the workplace is usually very directed; if the logistics of care provoke a physician to make changes, those changes, once made, usually alter the logistics of care. If patients stimulate a doctor to change, he or she is likely to change his or her interactions with patients.

CHANGES IN DIRECT PATIENT CARE

Forces for Change

We observed forty-nine changes affecting patient care. Physicians altered the way they took care of patients in response to one of three main types of influence arising in the clinical environment: Demand originating with the consumers of health-care–patients, assimilation of new information, and, least commonly, problems in the logistics of patient care.

Demand. In the clinical environment, patient demand was the influence most commonly cited as inducing change in the way care was given. "Demand," of course, has two connotations. As used by economists, the term describes the readiness to purchase goods or services. But demand also may be directly expressed as a desire for a specific intervention. For physicians, one implicit component of demand is the array of conditions they most often are asked to treat. Primary care physicians address a broad range of common but worrisome healthcare problems such as chronic fatigue, weight loss, chlamydia, or recurrent ear infections; whereas, subspecialists confine themselves to a more restricted range of conditions.

Demand includes not only the type of illness for which care is sought, but also the specific form of care that is offered. A urologist, for example, felt obliged to learn about nonoperative techniques for his patients with recurrent kidney stones, in order to provide appropriate and desirable care. In addition to the primarily *medical* elements of demand, there is often an explicitly economic component. For example, an internist noted that he was using less expensive drugs and ordering fewer investigations when he saw patients of poorer means.

Although demand is often tacit, patients also make open requests for a health-care service, for example, by calling for frank discussions of sexual problems or by asking for information on side effects of the drugs they receive. One family doctor acknowledged "giving patients what they want," that is, meeting the demands of an assertive and well-educated patient population. This kind of consumerism is prevalant among patients, who appear increasingly to be knowledgeable enough about diseases and treatments to request services more openly, and to ask for more frank disclosures of the costs and consequences of care.

Continuing education. To a degree that surprised us, many physicians attributed their changes to CME: after demand, it was the most frequently cited reason. The physicians' definition of CME was not confined to formal courses or planned activities, although such conferences or short courses were acknowledged as a significant influence for change. One physician, for example, attended a refresher course on common office problems and learned about the value of ordering a new serum iron test in the diagnosis of anemia. Information was also gleaned from less official but, nonetheless, planned activities, as was the case for a family physician practicing in a group that encouraged weekly teaching sessions with residents and staff physicians. Yet, for many, informal CME was mostly or entirely self-directed, and it exploited resources available in the clinical environment. These included standard journals as well as monographs and videotapes or audiotapes generated by drug companies.

Goldfinger (1982), among others, has called for a definition of CME broad enough to incorporate the variety of ways that useful learning occurs in the clinical environment: Hallway conversations, interactions with peers, discussions with consultants, or experiences with patients. These superficially haphazard interactions appeared to be a major source of learning for many, if not most, of the physicians we interviewed. This type of learning most often was applied to specific patient problems.

Of twelve broadly construed changes attributed directly to CME, three were derived from informal peer contact and three from reading journals. Several were occasioned by a combination of lectures and short courses, and one by formal consultation. No one reported making changes solely on the basis of information provided by people in other health professions, or by drug company representatives.

Logistics. The third, and least common, of the forces leading to changes in medical practices was attributed to logistics. One gastroenterologist, for example, changed his sigmoidoscopic technique when new equipment became available in his hospital.

Kinds of Change

Most changes affected use of equipment or procedures in diagnosis and treatment. Surprisingly few of the physicians interviewed indicated that they had changed their interview techniques to facilitate discussion of such important issues as sexuality or suicide potential. Changes in diagnostic practice predominated, and were made when physicians learned of newer procedures.

Changes made in response to the clinical environment were largely in the middle of the range of complexity and magnitude. Adjustments and redirections predominated to the extent that descriptions of change were consistent with the discrete typology developed for this analysis, although, in some cases, the distinctions were somewhat blurred. In direct patient care there were forty-nine changes, of which twenty-one were adjustments and twenty-three were redirections; only four were classified as accommodations, and one as a transformation.

Nearly one-third of the adjustments appeared to be stimulated by patient demand and affected treatment and follow-up. As a result of these changes, sexual problems were discussed more frankly, and informed consent procedures were made more explicit. Some laboratory tests were ordered more frequently in response to patients' expressed or implicit requirements. Fear about litigations also was used to support increased use of tests, but often was offset by concern about the cost of care for the poor.

The clinical environment itself served both as a stimulus to change patterns of patient care and as an instrument for education. Approximately one-third of such changes came about in response to information about new or better techniques of investigation or management. Information came from consultants, other peers, formal courses, journals and newsletters, and even the lay press. Often, new knowledge appeared not to emanate from a "point source," but to permeate the atmosphere. Rather than describing a particular source, physicians often reported that they learned about needed changes by "just hearing about them." Such common phrases as "I became aware" or "It was general knowledge" abounded. Whereas the response to patient demands tended to be somewhat generalized, new information was incorporated in relatively specific ways, for example, in the use of new, more sophisticated equipment, new diagnostic tests, or new medications. While most of these amounted to relatively minor shifts (such as the change from using a rigid sigmoidoscope to a flexible one), some of them were more substantial, for example, adopting of new nuclear imaging techniques.

Redirection was most probable when patients' problems were serious, and when the physician felt strongly identified with the anguish they caused. One family physician described how she began to alter the way she treated teenage maladjustment. She had visited a high school to lecture on the topic of depression and drug use, and while there, the funeral of a student who had committed suicide was announced. Both she and the students were deeply moved by the event and shaken by the coincidence. In the aftermath of this experience, she altered her protocol to include an in-depth assessment of suicide risk. In another example, a psychiatrist learned new, complex, and detailed psychotherapeutic skills when he was involved in intensive psychotherapy with a patient, also recalling a period of time when he himself had been in therapy.

Fewer than a third of redirections in the context of the clinical environment resulted from patient demand. In one case, an orthopedic surgeon gave in to patient requests that he inject chymopapain (an enzyme purported to chemically dissolve disc material) into lumbar discs rather than operate on them, although he felt that surgery was superior. Similarly, a plastic surgeon began applying permanent eye liner (a form of tattooing on the eyelid) after patients began to request the procedure. Other reasons for redirection, such as new information or a change in logistics, were rarely given.

There were only four changes classified as accommodations: they all reflected the physicians' own sense of coming to grips with, or feeling more comfortable with, a variety of problems in patient care. For example, two specialists in their early fifties said they were unhappy about, but resigned to, an increased number of problems arising from single parent families, including drug use, abuse of medical services, "nuisance calls," and other psychosocial problems for which they felt little could be done.

Only one transformation-type change was reported in patient care. A 42-year-old radiologist, when asked what had changed for him, said he was "sick and tired of [the practice of] medicine," and was making plans to leave it. His desire to leave healthcare was the result of increasing patient pressure and bureaucracy in medicine, which had prompted him to learn about the non-medical business world.

Learning

Although some physicians did no learning at all in making their changes, most employed a range of strategies, from highly informal to highly formal. Two specialists, possibly reflecting their sense of hopelessness in the face of psycho-social problems, made no effort to learn about them. A family physician, by contrast, learned how to deal with well-educated, assertive patients by talking with colleagues about their characteristics, and by sending for health information brochures. A general surgeon mastered a specific technique (surgery for colo-rectal cancer) that he could "claim as my own," using the deliberate, formal approach of attending appropriate workshops and courses to aid in accomplishing this task.

When the change was an adjustment, learning most often was directed toward specific problems, and acquired through formal CME. Physicians would respond to a clinical problem, a patient request, or something learned in the clinical context, with an explicit use of recognized resources—reading journals, texts, or monographs; formally consulting with a colleague; or attending courses or lectures. There were, however, several noteworthy exceptions to this general pattern. One family physician, finding that his patient population was becoming more and more pediatric in nature, devised and directed a conceptually-oriented program for himself by reviewing and taking notes from a general textbook of pediatrics. In other instances, resources were much less formal; physicians "heard" about new tests from colleagues, or took part in discussions about the specifics of new manual skills.

In the instances of redirection, learning approaches were more varied, even though the forces for change were more uniform. Most commonly, learning involved gaining experience related to a concrete problem, as was true when practices were adjusted. Very well-planned and more systematic approaches were used when dealing with screening procedures (e.g., routinely testing stools for occult blood, checking levels of dioxin in the workplace, or determining the risk of a specific virus infection in pregnancy). Also, informal resources for learning played a more important role when physicians described how they had "picked up" information about a new technology (e.g., the use of CAT scans in acoustic neuromas), or learned that a drug was no longer useful.

CHANGES IN THE LOGISTICS OF CARE

We recorded fifty-nine occasions of change in the logistics of patient care, eighteen percent more than in the content of patient care. Such changes affected the scheduling of office hours, moving or expanding office facilities, purchasing or using different equipment, and employing or relating to people in other health professions.

The physician's convenience, or efficiency in the use of time, motivated most of the logistics changes we recorded. An obstetrician wished to move closer to the hospital where his practice was centered; and a family practitioner chose to book all obstetric examinations on the same afternoon. Many physicians also reported the need to move from, or update, inadequate facilities. These changes, perceived as originating with the physician, accounted for twenty-five of the fifty-nine cases.

Patient demand was given as the reason for another twenty-three cases. An internist described moving his practice site because his elderly patients complained that he had no elevator in his building. Another opened his office one evening a week for commuters who could not attend a day clinic; and a plastic surgeon moved to a more elaborate office, feeling that his clientele "expected it." Physicians also adjusted referrals for diagnosis or consultation to accommodate their patients' requests. One rheumatologist initially referred patients requiring EMG's to the center where she had been trained, an hour's drive away. However, patients complained about the distance, so she began using a smaller but closer facility. If patient volume increased, measures to increase office or parking space had to be taken.

Alterations in patient demand also arose from shifts in the types of patients being seen. The most important influence was ability to pay. Less affluent patients waited until they were sicker to see the doctor. Once these patients were seen, physicians sometimes perceived themselves as having fewer options for treatment.

CME was cited as instrumental in only two logistic changes. As the result of suggestions given at a CME refresher course on psychiatry, one family physician began scheduling his counseling sessions at the end of the work day, when they could be more open-ended. A dermatologist developed a new filing system for reprints as the result of an article he had read on the "information explosion."

With logistics changes, it was apparent that while patient demands or patient volume were often at stake, physicians took considerable pleasure in directing their own affairs. They moved practice sites, or even changed practices in patient care with either or both a personal sense of relief and accomplishment. In contrast, accommodations to situations over which they felt no control were usually accompanied by negative emotions.

Types of Change

Most of the accommodations were a matter of accepting the inability of patients to pay for care. Economic limitations reduced the number of patients seen by a neurologist, a family physician, and a thoracic surgeon. When these doctors did see low-income patients, the patients were more likely to come in with serious illnesses.

Physicians also responded to their perceptions that patients are more likely than in the past to sue for malpractice. One thoracic surgeon, noting this tendency, claimed not to have altered his clinical practices as a result, although he was more aware of potential lawsuits, more detailed and careful in his note taking and management practices, and more defensive in his attitude. In almost all of these cases, the shift in attitude on the part of the physician was a negative one, expressed generally as "I don't like it, but what can I do?" Only one positive accommodation was noted, that by a physician who had an increase in patient volume as the economy picked up.

There were three major types of adjustment affecting the logistics of practice: (1) changes were made in office arrangements—personnel, schedules, or location of activities, (2) less frequently, diagnostic facilities, to which referrals were sent, were changed, and (3) in a few cases, the type of professional used for a certain function was changed (such adjustments affected the use of paramedics, emergency services, or consultants).

In the logistics of patient care, redirections were about as numerous as adjustments. Most frequent was moving an office, which was usually undertaken for the convenience of the patient and the physician and entailed fairly significant dislocations. Second in frequency was acquiring equipment, which might be either medical (a culposcope, CT scanner, NMR scanner, or apnea monitor), or managerial (an office computer system).

Learning

Change without learning, the simplest strategy for change, occurred in approximately a third of our cases and most often reflected negative, stoical acceptance of economic decline. Thus, physicians denied learning as they accepted losing patients, or terminated a component of practice (such as obstetrics). Change in the use of specialists as consultants also occurred without any acknowledged learning.

Sixteen of the physicians who did learn used an experiential problem-based strategy, and did so with about the same frequency, whether the change was an accommodation, adjustment, or redirection. For example, physicians prepared to deal with their perceptions that lawsuits were possible, or imminent, by consulting informally with lawyers, staff members, or other colleagues. In the process, they often would reorganize their notes or re-think a case.

Formal resources, such as CME courses or workshops, were used by thirteen other physicians who made more active kinds of change. Several physicians attended financial or investment seminars, run by private groups, as part of choosing to move offices, a process that often entailed buying land, buildings, or equipment.

More self-directed learning was reported in twelve cases. A neurologist who perceived that his group's patient load was decreasing learned marketing strategies by contacting knowledgeable persons in the field of health marketing.

Several family physicians and internists adjusting to varying patient loads (e.g., increasing numbers of geriatric patients), began to read, or attend more courses on relevant topics. A few physicians, taking new directions to accommodate pressures to change, employed a variety of formal and informal resources such as texts, literature searches, courses, and consultations. None of the learning strategies were directed toward gaining a general or conceptual understanding (the majority were geared toward solving a concrete problem).

Overall, most learning to produce change in the clinical environment was directed at a specific problem and was experiential in character. When the change to be made was an accommodation or, less likely, an adjustment, it often was made without learning, whereas most adjustments, and to a greater extent, re-directions almost always entailed learning. This sort of learning tended to be more deliberative and slightly more formal. The form that learning took usually seemed appropriate to its purpose—more deliberative when a complex, new theory or management technique was contemplated; more limited, formal, and problem-oriented when adjusting to a logistical situation or patient care practice.

Discussion

Changes made in relation to the clinical environment were virtually all adjustments or redirections, while perspective transformations and accommodations were virtually absent. In general, the larger changes were perceived as gratifying by the people who had made them. Accommodations were more likely to be accompanied by a negative tone—physicians acknowledged accepting more "hassles" from patients, or seeing fewer patients because of economic difficulties. The differences in response seemed to have little to do with the magnitude or nature of the problem, but rather with the physician's sense of being in control of the situation. The physicians' attitudes toward change or learning may have influenced their reactions as much as anything inherent in the situations.

The magnitude and complexity of active changes ranged from minor (substituting one antibiotic for another) to very large (moving offices, taking on a new research project, or dropping a major practice). Not surprisingly, the magnitude of change seemed to be correlated with the power or number of forces favoring it. Most changes affected treatment, fewer affected prognosis, and very few altered long-term follow-up, or examination and assessment skills. Perhaps this reflects the North American medical system's traditional emphasis on active diagnosis and treatment, rather than chronic illness and long-term care.

Learning Strategies and CME

The clinical environment presents a set of medical or logistical problems; solving them is an integral part of adapting to this environment. This reality supports the claim that problem-based learning is a keystone of physician education (Barrows and Tamblyn 1980). It also reflects ideas derived from adult learning theory (Tough 1971) that adults "use [learning] for taking action," often to deal with some task, situation, or activity.

CME was identified as both a contributor to change and a means to change. Physicians' definitions of CME were broad rather than narrow, and generally fell within the three categories developed by the Ontario Council for CME in 1980 (Williams, Bryans, and Davis 1981). *Formal* types of CME included planned educational opportunities, courses, traineeships, and medical meetings. *Informal* types were unplanned, readily accessible resources, such as texts, journals, audiotapes or videotapes, and monographs. Contextual or environmental types of CME were derived from clinical encounters, such as formal or informal consultations, or interactions with patients, other health professionals, and peers. Viewed from this broad perspective, CME becomes the learning arm of the clinical environment.

Coleman, Katz, and Menzel (1966), in their study of the adoption of a new drug among physicians, delineate two kinds of information sources: Those which initiate change (such as a patient or pharmaceutical salesman), and those which legitimize it. Our data supports this bifold function of CME. Through CME, physicians may become aware of a practice that might be changed, and after interpretation and internalization of this information, change may occur without any further learning or action. In our cases, most of these changes emerged from the logistics of practice, fewer from direct patient care.

In legitimizing change, CME may operate to alter perceptions of the need or potential for change. For example, a physician may hear about a new weight-loss program through a colleague or a patient, but be reluctant to learn more about it because of lack of time or a sense of futility in dealing with obese patients. In such an instance, CME may enable the physician to see that these patients can be helped. Finally, CME resources may be used in their well-recognized and traditional roles: To assist physicians in reinterpreting and reinforcing what they have learned, thus easing implementation of different practices.

Several recommendations about the structure and function of CME flow from our observations of the clinical environment. First, to be effective for the real-life problems encountered by physicians, CME must rely not only on presentation of concepts and diseases, but also should integrate problem-centered learning. Problem-based learning and problem solving are key elements of the practicing physician's learning strategies. CME must mimic and support this process. Although the value of problem-based learning has been supported by empirical research, and although it is being incorporated into the undergraduate curricula of many medical schools, formal CME programs still rely heavily on lectures. This may, in part, explain why CME programs have so little influence (Bertram and Brooks-Bertram 1977; Lloyd and Abrahamson 1979; Stein 1981).

Second, our data supports the inclusion of continuing education modalities that cross traditional boundaries into the clinical environment. Such programs can be established through peer review activities, audit and feedback procedures, and ward or clinic rounds. The clinical environment creates a plethora of influences favoring change. The reality is that these influences are neither "purely" medical nor "purely" logistical. An integrated approach could lead to better healthcare, and perhaps to greater efficiency.

Finally, CME no longer may be confined, either by definition or practice, to a rigid framework of formal, or even informal, courses or resources. It must, to be effective, be seen as a contextual process, involving peers, colleagues, and indeed, most of the human elements of the environment.

In summary, for the sake of patients, and as a responsibility of educators, healthcare providers, administrators, or policymakers, the concepts of learning and change, and the components of the clinical environment must be brought together. CME of a formal or informal variety must be at least practice-oriented, or optimally, practice-based; contextual learning must be probed and facilitated; and learning must be introduced firmly and solidly into the everyday clinical environment—to be internalized by the physician and institutionalized by the system.

REFERENCES

Barrows, H. S., and P. Tamblyn. 1980. *Problem-based learning: An approach to medical education*. New York: Springer-Verlag.

Bertram, D. A., and P. A. Brooks-Bertram. 1971. The evaluation of continuing medical education: A literature review. *Health Education Monographs* 5:330–348.

Coleman, J. S., E. Katz, and H. Menzel. 1966. *Medical innovations—A diffusive study*. Indianapolis: Bobbs-Merrill.

Davis, D., et al. 1984. The Impact of CME: A methodological review of continuing medical education literature. *Evaluation and the Health Professions* 7:251–283.

Goldfinger, S. E. 1982. Continuing medical education: The case for contamination. *New England Journal of Medicine* 306:540–541.

Lloyd, J. S., and S. Abrahamson. 1979. The effectiveness of continuing medical education: A review of the evidence. *Evaluation and the Health Professions* 2:251–280.

Stein, L. S. 1981. Effectiveness of continuing medical education: Eight research reports. *Journal of Medical Education* 56:103–110.

Sweet, R. L. 1988. Pelvic inflammatory disease: Prevention and treatment. *Modern Medicine of Canada* 43:345–350.

Tough, A. 1971. *The Adult's Learning Projects*. Toronto: Ontario Institute for Studies in Evaluation. (6).

Williams, J. I., A. M. Bryans, and D. A. Davis. 1981. The continuing medical education of physicians in Ontario: Practices, needs and problems. *Ontario Council on CME: Report*. Toronto: University of Toronto Press.

8

Relationships with Medical Institutions

Jocelyn M. Lockyer and John Parboosingh

I was surprised when I was appointed Chief of Surgery two months ago.
The job is not too onerous—I have to conduct staff meetings, report minutes,
serve on the executive commitee of the hospital, and work out a few problems
in the operating room. Over the past two months, I have spoken to the
previous Chief of Surgery, Head of the Operating Room, and Hospital
Administrator about the job. I also read the hospital by-laws.

I have been interested in substance abuse since I finished my residency
in psychiatry. When my hospital decided to open up a Substance Abuse
Center eighteen months ago, the Director of Mental Health Services asked
me if I wanted to be the medical director. I agreed, but it has been a big
change. I spend hours attending meetings and doing paperwork. Since I had
not seen very many substance abusers in two years, I had to do some
updating. I subscribed to several new journals. I have gone to eight courses
in six states, lasting from a day to a week. I also visited fifteen treatment
centers.

Hospitals, clinics, and medical schools have become important affiliations for
physicians. Contemporary diagnosis, investigation, and treatment requires that
physicians consult with medical colleagues in different specialties, use equipment
available only to groups of physicians, and involve other health professionals in
the delivery of patient care services (Moss et al. 1966). Such affiliations are
increasing as, "A 1984 American Hospital Association survey revealed that
seventy percent of responding hospitals had medical staff members on their
boards, filling 22.7 percent of the voting positions" (Cohn 1986, 58). The same

survey stated that whereas four percent of hospitals reported compensating physicians for administrative responsibilities in 1973, by 1984, forty-one percent of hospitals provided full or part-time compensation to at least one physician for administrative duties. The average hospital employed 3.9 physicians (Morrisey and Brooks 1985). Similarly, group practices in clinics have become more attractive, and the groups are becoming larger and more diversified (Kralewski, Pitt, and Shatin 1985).

In eighty-six of the cases of change reported by fifty-three physicians, the association with an institution was described as the wellspring of change. The changes varied from assuming a formal administrative appointment or committee responsibility, to developing new clinical skills to enable a move to other institutions. Learning was an integral part of the change process, although both the quantity and intensity of learning varied. Modest learning was described when the hospital rather than the physician, was the primary benefactor of the change, for example, chairing a committee. Conversely, substantive and prolonged learning was associated with adopting new procedures, for example, cardiac catheterization in support of a new service for the institution.

The function of this chapter is to report and analyze changes in which the institutions with which the physicians were associated (namely hospitals, medical schools, and medical centers) were the primary cause of change. The reasons for change are examined, the types of change are categorized, and the relationship between the reasons and the types of change are described. The role of learning in the change process is also described and discussed. Finally, some implications for hospitals, medical schools, and clinics are offered.

REASONS FOR CHANGE WITHIN INSTITUTIONS

The process of change was often different, based upon the presence or absence of certain characteristics of the physicians and the institutional settings. Six factors related to the qualities of individual physicians and their institutional milieus were evident. How and what kind of change was made depended on:

1. The presence of significant *previous experience* related to an institutional role

2. Whether change was necessary in order to serve as a *member of a team*

3. The extent to which the change represented a valued but *unsolicited opportunity*

4. The chance for the physician's *professional/career opportunities* to be promoted

5. The potential for the development of *new patient care programs* in the institution

6. The presence of *interpersonal conflict* within the institution

Previous experience, including experience on committees, administrative appointments, or the possession of unique skills, was offered as a principle reason for over one-third (30) of the changes. An appointment to a hospital staff carries with it the expectation that, in addition to serving patients, the physician will participate in quality assurance activities; teach other physicians, medical students, and other health professionals; and develop new programs and services. New members of a medical staff will normally be assigned to one or two minor committees, usually based on their experience. ''When physicians are recognized as 'competent, honest, and well organized' by their colleagues and other professionals, they begin to receive requests to participate in [other] committees, programs, and projects or may be given a formal managerial position'' (Ruelas and Leatt 1985, 156). Two physicians described how their experiences became a reason for changes in their activities. A psychiatrist reported that he had taken on the task of running a family therapy conference for residents, which he saw as a natural next step from the family therapy course he had taught to nursing students. Similarly, a gastroenterologist became associate medical director in his hospital, after serving for eleven years as chief of internal medicine. Both of the examples cited show the progressive nature of the responsibilities that physicians assume in conjunction with their primary tasks of providing patient care in the institution.

In nineteen of the changes, physicians perceived that their responsibilities as *members of a team* were important reasons for change, placing the goals of the institution before their personal goals. Institutional priorities encouraged the physicians to alter patterns of work to accommodate students, acquire new skills, or even to change ways of thinking about the job. For example, a physician in the military stated that when he was promoted to department chairman, he realized that his prior experience had not equipped him for his new responsibilities. He ''needed help to become a good department chairman.'' Consequently, he attended a two-week course on management skills for senior physicians. In another case, the physician agreed to serve on his hospital's medical advisory committee. He stated, ''It is part of citizenship.''

As colleagues within an institution alter their responsibilities, *unsolicited opportunities*, including new roles and positions, are created for others. For example, a young general surgeon reported surprise at his appointment as chief of surgery, as he had not actively sought this position, but saw it as an opportunity. At the request of his hospital board, a senior internist was appointed president of a community health service agency following a crisis in which most of the board had resigned. Unsolicited opportunities such as these provided the stimulus for change in eleven of these cases.

Career aspirations were the reason for change in thirteen cases. One physician indicated that he did his best to force his own appointment as director of diagnostic radiology at his university. He interviewed for positions at other institutions, knowing it would ''get back'' to his dean that he was looking elsewhere.

The development of *new programs* by institutions, demanding new medical skills, such as coronary angioplasty or nuclear imaging, was the main stimulus to change in six cases. Physicians had to modify their work patterns to provide the new services. In some cases, instead of stimulating the learning of a new skill, new hospital directions resulted in the redirection of an activity. The

Table 8.1
Types of Changes and Learning Activities

		No Learning	Learning	Total
I	Accommodation	17	13	30
II	Adjustment	10	22	32
III	Redirection	5	16	21
IV	Transformation	0	3	3
Total		32	54	86

development of a neonatal intensive care unit staffed by salaried neonatologists stimulated a 62-year-old pediatrician to discontinue his neonatal practice.

Not all physicians work effectively in a group environment (Georgopoulos and Mann 1962). *Interpersonal conflict* between physicians of different specialties, between older and younger physicians, and between salaried and attending physicians can initiate change. While relatively infrequent, the conflict may be substantive enough to cause a radical change for the individual and the organization. In five of the six cases of change triggered by interpersonal conflict, the physician left the organization. A pediatric gastroenterologist recalled that a new director was appointed to his unit. "I did not see eye to eye with him . . . this was very traumatic." As a consequence he left the hospital where he had been working for five years. In a second case, an emergency room physician stated that he did not approve of many of the cost-cutting policies instituted by a new administrator, so he moved. Such examples demonstrate the powerful impact on the physician and on the institution that interpersonal tension can have.

Each of these six triggers can be associated primarily with either the interests of the physician or his institution. Changes triggered by previous experience, the requirements of team membership, and unsolicited opportunites were usually associated with the needs of the institution. The physician's career aspirations, new hospital programs, and interpersonal conflicts, although functions of institutional relationships, more often reflected the individual needs of physicians. These triggers were also more frequently associated with greater effort by the physician in making a change. Closer inspection of the types of change and learning activities revealed some of the ways these factors affected the overall process of change.

TYPES OF CHANGES AND LEARNING

Accommodations, adjustments, redirections, and transformations were described by our subjects as effects of their different kinds of relationships in medical institutions. (See table 8.1.) The smaller accommodations, and adjustment changes, occurred most frequently, accounting for seventy-two percent of the changes. Redirection changes accounted for another quarter of the changes. There were only three transformations reported.

Learning was an integral part of the change process in most instances. The most prolonged and intense learning occurred with the more substantive changes. Most redirections and all three of the perspective transformations involved learning. Conversely, small changes involved less learning, and over one-half of accommodations did not involve learning. Overall, physicians stated learning had not occurred in one-third of the cases (32 out of 86).

Accommodations were rarely sought by the physicians for themselves. Those usually involved little effort. More than half (55 percent) of accommodation changes were accomplished without new learning efforts, since most believed that their previous experience and training had qualified them for their new roles or activities.

In contrast, adjustments demanded more thought in order to make the alteration in daily activities, even though the change often was small. A child psychiatrist, for example, stated that he wanted the position of assistant training director. He spent about forty hours discussing his responsibilities with the director, directors of other programs, and other hospital and university staff before taking the job, although the job itself required only approximately four hours each week. Learning was more prevalent in adjustment changes compared with accommodations, and occurred about two-thirds of the time.

In contrast to smaller, simpler changes, redirections of major elements of life or practice were fewer, but required more effort over longer periods. They more often were associated with learning even though they accounted for slightly fewer than one-quarter of all the changes caused by institutional roles. A pathologist, for example, described why he moved from a full-time medical faculty position to a new hospital setting as chairman of the laboratories department. He had served as acting head of his department at the university for eighteen months. The dean of the faculty decided to bring in a new chairman. The new head "was a researcher who had not had any clinical or administrative experience." The pathologist had the option of waiting it out and engaging in "academic guerrilla warfare," or alternately, he could leave, which he did. A second physician, trained in public health administration, bitterly complained that she was fired as head of one state program, but had applied for and received the directorship of another program. Her new appointment caused her to refocus her career and aspirations. In preparation for the new position, she attended several training sessions and workshops and did a lot of reading. Both of these examples demonstrate the substantive nature of redirection changes that result in an altered workday and often a new working environment. Learning activities were involved in three-quarters of redirections. For the majority of the physicians, research and consultation with friends and colleagues were integral parts of the change process.

Transformation changes were the largest and most complicated changes. In perspective transformations, a major philosophical metamorphosis was also associated with the restructuring of life or practice. Reorganization, redefinition, and reinterpretation of fundamental beliefs and experiences based on new principles and meanings were required. Three such transformations were described,

Table 8.2
The Types of Change and the Stimuli for Change

	I Accom	II Adjust	III Redir	IV Transfor	Total
Experience	16	9	3	2	30
Opportunity	7	2	2	0	11
Team	5	12	1	1	19
Career	1	7	5	0	13
Programs	0	2	5	0	7
Conflict	1	0	5	0	6
Total	30	32	21	3	86

all involving substantial learning projects. For example, a general surgeon agreed to spend ninety percent of his time as medical director of his health maintenance organization (HMO). As one member of his small clinic of seventeen physicians, he had attended a meeting of the American Academy of Medical Directors where he heard a discussion about HMO's. He then attended a workshop on HMO's in another state a year later and came home convinced that his small group practice would function as an HMO in almost an ideal fashion. In spite of considerable resistance from colleagues, he persisted, and two years later his clinic became the first HMO in his state. Between his first conceptualization of an HMO and the establishment of his HMO four years later, he read extensively and brought in consultants. In the process, he discovered and joined the Group Health Association of America, which led him to many educational sessions and seminars and site visits to several facilities. This example demonstrates a change that was more than a change from surgeon to medical administrator. The surgeon underwent a profound attitudinal and philosophical change in his beliefs about the delivery of healthcare.

Physicians described all four types of change—accommodation, adjustment, redirection, and perspective transformation—as consequences of their relationships with medical institutions. Learning was an essential process for change in two-thirds of the cases, but learning activities varied from modest to substantial. The most intensive learning activities were associated with the most substantive changes. Conversely, learning rarely was required for modest changes. If the change was small and the physician felt a previous experience was the essential prerequisite to the new role, he rarely undertook learning activities, and certainly none that required much time.

FORCE FOR CHANGE AND TYPES OF CHANGE

In understanding the force of the institution in the physician's life, it is important to examine the stimuli for change in conjunction with the types of change. Very distinct patterns occur. (See table 8.2.) Previous experience and unsolicited opportunity most frequently were associated with accommodation changes. Adjustments were found in conjunction with the requirements of being a team player and career aspirations. Interpersonal conflict and the development of new programs most likely were to be associated with redirections.

Over half of accommodations were the result of the physician's previous experience. Unsolicited opportunities and team membership accounted for another third. One physician described his appointment to the infection control committee of his hospital that met once a month. He did not perceive that his appointment had depended on any particular expertise he had. He did a minimal amount of extra reading, when first appointed, and occasionally read in specific areas when an item on the agenda required preparation. Such an example is indicative of how physicians accept hospital generated responsibilities that are not of particular interest to them, and consequently, expend minimal energy to meet these obligations.

Adjustment changes, which required a more thoughtful modification of behavior, were associated with team membership in one-third of the cases. However, previous experience and career aspirations were also important. For example, a specialist in infectious diseases recognized there was a need to develop a clinical service in infectious diseases at his hospital. To this end, he began accepting undergraduate students for elective rotations, soliciting consultations in infectious diseases for teaching purposes, and spending a considerable amount of time generating proposals for funding, so that a fellowship program in infectious disease could begin. In this case, the physician modified his work toward his new goal after considering the benefits to his hospital.

Adding, dropping, or substituting major areas of endeavor, characteristic of redirections, most often were associated with interpersonal conflicts, the development of new patient care programs, and physicians' career aspirations (3 of 4 cases). For most redirections, individual goals and priorities played a more substantive role than did institutional goals. A pediatric gastroenterologist described how, following a personality clash with the new director, he left the hospital he had been affiliated with for five years to develop a general pediatric practice without hospital privileges. In preparation for the change, he had to read more and attended review courses in general pediatrics. This is an example of how a physician can drop an activity and substitute a new set of activities geared toward the enhancement of new goals.

Generally, smaller, simpler changes (accommodations and adjustments) usually were stimulated by the physician's previous experience, the responsibilities of team membership, and unsolicited opportunities. Normally, such changes required little effort on the part of the physician, and institutional priorities (rather than the physician's personal goals) were most important. Redirection changes more often were stimulated by the development of new programs by the institution, by interpersonal conflict, and by career aspirations. In many of these examples cited, the physician's personal ambitions overrode the benefits the institution might accrue, and the physician exerted much greater energy than he would have for a change in which the institution was the primary benefactor.

FORCES FOR CHANGE AND LEARNING

More energies were expended by physicians in making some changes than in others. Generally, the more complicated the change and the greater the personal benefit to the physician, the more effort was used in thinking about and carrying out the necessary learning activities in the change process. Learning activities were reported eighty-five percent of the time when the change was stimulated by either the establishment of new programs or by interpersonal conflict. For six of the seven changes that were stimulated by the development of new patient care programs, the learning involved intensive educational activities, including apprenticeships, short courses, discussions with colleagues, and reading.

Learning activities were not so prevalent when other stimuli were at work. For changes involving unsolicited opportunities, learning was reported as being instrumental in the change process less than one-third of the time. Changes that benefited the institution rather than the individual often involved little learning. An examination of the thirty-two changes in which the physicians did not report any learning indicated that three-quarters of them were minor changes involving a reassignment of time, new committee responsibility, or the end of a term of office. As Ruelas and Leatt (1985) identified, physicians acting in administrative roles, and who do not have formal preparation in administration, tend to learn what to do through observation of others who have held the position. The role models are most likely to be other physician executives and professional ad-ministrators with whom they work, and the learning process is often one of trial and error rather than thoughtful, purposeful pursuit of knowledge and skill.

LEARNING STRATEGIES

When institutional roles and relationships caused change, learning directed toward solving a practical problem was more common (72.2 percent of cases) than learning directed toward a more general, conceptual understanding. The solving of specific problems was the most common learning objective of phy-sicians who were taking new directions or making adjustments in their lives or practices. An ophthalmologist described how he had been a full-time member of a university faculty and ran a very successful service program monitoring eye changes in preterm infants. Unfortunately, as the demand for his program had grown, the funding for personnel and equipment had not kept up, causing him considerable frustration. He had several fruitless meetings with his department head over a two-year period that finally culminated in a meeting with his dean. The dean reaffirmed the department head's statement that additional funding would not be available. The dean further stated that if the ophthalmologist did not see his future in the university, he should go into private practice. The ophthalmologist consulted a financial advisor who helped him assess his potential income in private practice. After six months of deliberation, he left the university.

This "problem as a focal point" approach was quite typical of those who encountered concrete problems within their institutions.

Deliberating and reflecting about alternatives rather than engaging in direct experiences was the learning method in sixty-one percent of the changes. However, for those who were making certain types of changes, an experiential approach, such as trying out a committee chairmanship, would not have been a reasonable way to learn how to perform a particular role. A psychiatrist appointed to the chair of the ethics committee of her state's psychiatric society employed a typical strategy in her attempt to handle the issues involved with the responsibility; she weighed the pros and cons as she talked to her colleagues and studied materials supplied by the national society on ethics. Experiential approaches, however, generally were used in conjunction with the development of new skills, particularly those that were gradually learned by using a large number of different resources over an extended period.

Formal learning resources, that is, materials, persons, or programs officially sanctioned for their value in learning, were more common (62.9 percent) than were informal resources. All transformations relied to a larger extent on formal resources. The surgeon who had become head of his HMO (and came to believe that HMOs were the optimal method of delivering patient care) engaged in a number of learning activities—reading, conferences, consultations with experts on HMOs, tours of HMOs, and membership in the Group Health Association of America. The use of formal resources is not surprising. As Ruelas and Leatt (1985) comment, physician executives tend to make use of skills and values that were previously associated with and shaped by their clinical roles. Their training has taught them to solve problems through a meticulous, analytical approach to decison making. Information obtained from recognized textbooks and professors will be perceived as more beneficial than information gained through informal means.

SUMMARY AND CONCLUSIONS

Physicians and their institutions have strong and symbiotic relationships. The patterns that emerged when the institution was the primary force in effecting the change were as follows:

1. Previous experience and team membership were the most important stimuli for changes. Institutions require that their medical staffs assume responsibilities for teaching, quality assurance, and other activities as part of the terms of membership. In exchange for these voluntary, usually unremunerated activities, physicians are assured their patients will be well-cared-for according to certain minimum standards.

2. The majority of changes were small-scale accommodations or adjustments. They were minor modifications of a physician's activity within his institution. Generally they did not have an economic impact on the physician. Institutional, rather than personal priorities, predominated. The time involved was minimal, and few modifications to

the work schedule were ever necessary, as physicians agreed to serve on committees, finished terms of office, or accepted minor administrative positions.

3. Physicians' personal priorities and ambitions were evident when they undertook changes that required major reorganizations of their work and concomitant intensive learning projects.

4. Learning was a primary means for making two-thirds of the changes. Learning activities were particularly important for large changes (e.g., redirections and perspective transformations), especially when the changes were stimulated by interpersonal conflicts or by the development of new programs or services. In such cases, personal gains were placed before institutional goals. Learning was rarely described for changes involving an unsolicited opportunity, and when it was described, the information source was usually limited to a colleague or the previous incumbent in the job.

5. Physicians most frequently selected learning strategies directed toward solving tangible problems, formal resources, and deliberative methods. In doing this, they fell back on their medical training, that encouraged observation, formally endorsed resources, and an analytical approach to decison making.

IMPLICATIONS AND DISCUSSION

In their formal relationships with medical institutions, physicians not only filled roles as healthcare providers but also as administrators of clinical services and as committee members. However, few physicians will spend the time required to develop administrative skills. Most seemed to agree that the long-term effectiveness of a physician functioning in an institution is dependent on his clinical, not administrative, acumen. Nonetheless, as hospital programs and the provision of care have become more complex, hospitals and other medical institutions are increasing the demands they make on physicians to assist with clinical and administrative planning and decision making.

Physicians who perceive personal benefits accruing from work done on behalf of these institutions seem to be more likely to use greater amounts of energy to change, and to spend more time in formal and informal learning activities. On the other hand, when the greatest benefit seems to be for the hospital, the physician is less likely to be as active in pursuit of the change. Administrators, in planning changes in hospital services or requesting volunteers for committees, should be cognizant of the need to make efficacious use of physicians' time. Work assigned must be meaningful, and careful selection of interested physicians is critical to the success of most projects.

Institutions must take a role in helping physicians perform administrative duties well. Most physicians acquire administrative skills by serving as a member of committees. Early in the process, their colleagues serve as their primary sources of information and skill development (Ruelas and Leatt 1985). Role modeling is an excellent way to learn the skills of serving effectively on a committee; however, by the time a physician is appointed to a middle management position, some administrative training is usually necessary. Short courses conducted by management experts in a "peer learning" situation have been found to be particularly helpful. For physician administrators at the department head level, courses should be supplemented by reading, and in some cases, by an affliation with professional organizations. A formal administrative degree will be of help to the physician who aspires to a senior administrative position in government or a major teaching institution, where his clinical expertise will be secondary to his administrative skill.

Large hospitals, management schools in conjunction with medical schools, and professional organizations have roles to play in ensuring the effectiveness of physicians serving in administrative capacities. They can develop orientation programs for new members of the medical staff and educational programs for medical staff leadership, as well as the traditional continuing professional education programs (Williams and Donnelly 1982). Management schools, in conjunction with medical schools or medical organizations, should continue to develop and improve educational programs for physicians in medical administration. The professional organizations that currently exist to upgrade the administrative expertise of physicians should continue their efforts to develop educational courses and materials. Often, there is lag-time between the assumption of major administrative responsibilities and the time physicians learn about medical management courses. Medical schools, through their CME offices, might serve as information brokers to assist physicians, newly appointed to administrative positions, in the selection of appropriate courses.

In summary, almost fifteen percent of the physicians who participated in the study described conditions in relationships with medical institutions as primary forces for change. Six factors were discussed—the physicians' previous experience, the institutions' requirements for team membership, the physicians' professional or career aspirations, unsolicited opportunities, the development of new patient care programs, and interpersonal conflicts. When the change was a modest one, the institution rather than the individual physician was usually perceived to be the primary beneficiary, and little or no learning was involved. Changes in which the physicians benefited more than the institution were most often large and complex ones requiring extensive learning characterized by a focus on specific problems, deliberative methods, and formal resources.

REFERENCES

Cohn, R. E. 1986. The medical director—the untapped potential of the position. *Hospital and Health Services Administration* 31(6):51–61.

Georgopoulos, B. S., and F. C. Mann. 1962. *The community general hospital.* New York: Macmillan.

Kralewski, J. E., L. Pitt, and D. Shatin. 1985. Structural characteristics of medical group practices. *Administrative Science Quarterly* 30:34–45.

Morrisey, M. A., and D. C. Brooks. 1985. Physician influence in hospitals: An update. *Hospital* (September):86–89.

Moss, A. B., et al. 1966. *Hospital Policy Decisions: Process and Action*. New York: G. P. Putnam's Sons.

Ruelas, E., and P. Leatt. 1985. The roles of physician executives in hospitals: A framework for management education. *Journal of Health Administration Education* Spring, 3(2, pt. 1):151–169.

Williams, K. J., and P. R. Donnelly. 1982. *Medical care quality and the public trust*. Chicago: Pluribus Press.

9

Relating to Others in the Profession

Harold A. Paul and Charles E. Osborne

As a therapeutic radiologist, I have been treating cancer patients for about twenty years. I'm proud to say that the hospital where I work is committed to the latest and best in cancer diagnosis and treatment.

A few months ago, three surgeons appeared in my office. We know each other well. They are in separate practices, but each of them has been sending me patients who need radiation treatment for cancer. Together, we have treated many patients. Furthermore, we all like to go to the weekly Tumor Conference to present and discuss other complicated cancer cases.

The surgeons asked me to start a program of intra-operative irradiation for patients with pancreatic cancer. They had read an article that described good results. Up to now, as any doctor knows, the science of medicine has had poor results in treating this form of cancer.

I was convinced. I had been reading too. I know the clinical team that did the original work reported in the article. We belong to the same national societies. They are honest, and they do good work.

This is how I went about it. First, I called up a radiologist at a first-rate medical school fifty miles away. He is also on the medical staff of a major hospital in that city. He came out and spent several hours going over the subject with me and with the surgeons. Next, because he had treated so many patients, I contacted an author of the original article. When he visited us, I made it a point to quiz him on many technical details.

We worked out an efficient patient management protocol with the cancer surgeons. I helped to write a set of procedures for the operating room nurses and presented it to them in a series of in-service training sessions. Our first case went without a hitch. I was pleased, and so were all of my professional colleagues.

Physicians live and work in relationships with one another. They form complex networks generating powerful forces both for change and for stability. In our sample, sixty-six episodes of change were ascribed to relationships with other physicians—singly, as with a consultant, partner, or colleague, or collectively, as with a professional society, peers in a hospital, or practice organization. The large majority (54 changes) were in the context of a group: a professional society (21), a partnership group (16), an informal hospital group (14), or a group of peers not defined in any clear way (3). The remaining twelve instances of change were ascribed to a relationship with one other physician. Differences can be seen between those changes concerning relationships between one physician and another as well as changes that involve a physician's relationship with a group.

CONSULTANTS AND MENTORS: INDIVIDUAL AGENTS OF CHANGE

All the changes arising from one doctor's relationship with another took place in the context of a *consultation*—broadly defined as any directed and purposeful exchange of information between two doctors for the benefit of patients. Consultations were either formal, in that a patient was referred and billed for the service, or informal, in that the patient was not charged and may have been described rather than seen. Without exception, the changes resulting from consultation involved strategies for patient care.

Consultations are key channels in medicine for the diffusion of technological innovation, and they are stimuli for change. Although it is conventionally thought of as a specific request for a specialist's input, often a consultation is between two physicians of the same specialty and roughly comparable levels of training, as when one neurologist calls another for advice before prescribing calcium-channel blockers for a migrane headache. In a more common pattern of response, one surgeon, for example, may decide to change his approach to breast cancer after observing a partner's practice and querying colleagues ouside the partnership. The key feature of consultation is the accumulation of pertinent new information from colleagues whose opinions are respected.

Consulting relationships between individual physicians led to change in a variety of ways. Sometimes a single conversation with a partner led to the introduction of a new drug in the doctor's practice. Other times, there was a series of conversations relating to a single change. That series could be with the same person, with several, or with a group identified with the innovation. When a major change, such as the introduction of a complex, new surgical procedure, was being planned, formal consultation with a group was more likely but often was supplemented by several informal consultations.

There are times when one physician, usually a partner, may serve another as a mentor or tutor for months or years. The mentor relationship is identified by Levinson (1978) as one of the most important a person can have in early adulthood. He characterizes a mentor as someone older than the subject, by 8–15 years, who serves as an advisor, teacher, sponsor, and more. A mentor may also be a guide who introduces the subject to a new world and to new people. Or the mentor may be an exemplar, someone who supports and facilitates "the realization of a dream." Levinson's basis for this description was an investigation of development and change in forty men. All were (nonmedical) professionals between the ages of thirty-five and forty-five.

In our sample, perhaps because the subjects tended to be older than Levinson's, no mentor was found who met all his criteria. However, there were two examples of significant learning and change that were caused by a sustained association with a partner. In one particularly striking example, the mentor was younger but otherwise corresponded exactly with Levinson's concept. A 60-year-old pediatrician described how a younger partner, skilled in the care of newborns and premature babies, had joined his group several years before. The competence of the younger partner was impressive. He was a model of a continuing student, always learning, always checking and validating his knowledge and professional competence. Because of this younger partner, the older physician was introduced to specific experts at the academic medical center and came to know them personally. He learned from his younger colleague how to find the most useful medical literature and where to attend the most beneficial conferences. He said that he considered his younger partner to be a "special stimulus to learning." Eventually, the younger doctor left the group. When that happened, the older physician then described himself as motivated to assume the primary responsibility for all neonatal care within the practice group, a responsibility that had formerly belonged to his younger partner. He continued to learn through attending conferences, reading, and staying in touch with his former young mentor. The distinction between a consultant and a mentor is not necessarily a sharp one. This case could be characterized as a sustained and complex consultant relationship, but it seems closer to the mark to call it mentoring. That there were only two such relationships identified in our sample is, perhaps, not surprising, since consultation is a great deal more common than mentoring.

INFORMAL GROUPS

Peer Pressure

Ill-defined as it may be, informal "peer pressure" can be a real force for change. Physicians in our sample sometimes planned detailed and complex learning projects that not only depended in an important way on the skills, support, and good will of their colleagues, but also were instigated by observing the practice of respected colleagues.

A 42-year-old ophthalmologist first became aware of a new operation by reading scientific articles and attending national conferences. Although he was really quite satisfied with his current procedures, he decided to change, in part because he began to notice a marked increase in the number of ophthalmologists in his community who were instituting the newer procedure. He defined this influence as "covert peer pressure." He described how he inferred the trend from his colleagues' behavior, and how he used them to learn this new procedure. After first studying the literature and reviewing videotapes at the local medical school, he scheduled his time so he could observe and question individual colleagues, on fifteen different occasions, as they performed the new procedure. As a final step, he asked a trusted friend, another ophthalmologist, to scrub with him on his first case.

"Covert peer pressure" may also be experienced as a negative, even hostile force. One primary physician described a defensive step he took when he began to feel that other physicians in his community were giving early stages of prenatal care, and then leaving the patient in her last trimester to arrange for care with a physician who could hospitalize for delivery. He regarded this as an insensitive practice that, in effect, resulted in abandoning patients. In response, he instituted a policy that he would accept no new obstetrical patients in his practice. He would care only for former patients.

A surgeon said that his peers had assessed him as overly aggressive—"knife happy," in his words. They also believed that his patients sustained too many complications. His response was to change practice location to another community, and to change to another specialty.

In these two cases, the "other" physicians were not an organized, formally defined group. The "generalized" group of peers was seen as either forming a negative judgment or exerting a negative influence over one aspect of the physician's practice. Although there were only three such instances, in two of three the change tended to be defensive, so as to evade the effect of the group action.

Hospital Colleagues

Hospitals are fertile ground for a variety of changes because they are an important part of the daily practice of many physicians. Hospitals bring together partners and competitors. In addition, they bring together practitioners of many of the twenty-three specialties, plus numerous sub-specialties, that collectively make up the fabric of modern medicine.

Within the hospital environment many official roles link doctor to doctor, and the doctors to others in the hospital organization, as discussed in Chapter Eight. However, informal relationships are more numerous and very influential. These informal groups often are temporary and without official status, as was true of the surgeons in our introductory case, who joined together to articulate the need for a new treatment method. The stimuli from these informal groups usually are seen positively, but sometimes they are viewed as negative forces for change, as when a pediatric surgeon described his continuing and fruitless debate with a clinical department regarding the relationship of pediatricians to surgeons, and the quality of residency training programs. In contrast, a primary physician, responding to a clearly changing viewpoint among his peers, learned how to alter his practice patterns by admitting fewer patients and performing more outpatient procedures. In another example, an anesthesiologist responded to the collective appeal, first from obstetricians, then from thoracic surgeons, to institute a new form of epidural anesthesia. These groups serve as a key force for change.

FORMAL GROUPS

The Partnership

Physicians in a partnership sometimes might respond to each other as consultants, but partners as a group sometimes also acted to bring about change. Of sixteen such changes, nine affected the business side of a group's medical practice. Examples included decisions to participate in certain health insurance plans, decisions about ownership of facilities, and the retirement of a senior partner. In one case, there was a decision to substitute a new form of treatment because of the partnership's concern over medicare reimbursement regulations.

Professional (Medical) Organizations

Approximately one-third of the changes (21 of 66) involved physicians in professional organizations. The kind of change described was determined largely by the nature and scope of the particular organization. The change was either directed toward maintenance of the organization itself, or it may have influenced the welfare of patients, usually in groups. For example, the purposes of a small society for hospital epidemiologists may be to publish a journal and hold an annual meeting. Such activities will produce constructive change in patient care through education and improved discourse among society members. A national organization for pediatricians may review immunization procedures, decide on the best current methods, and publish that information. The health of many will benefit as pediatricians take steps to follow new recommendations. Other organizations may work actively to influence legislation, for example, by working on new laws for travel safety. Many associations develop codes of ethics and revise them periodically. Others facilitate clinical research, or provide well-edited materials for patient education. Organizations also engage in activities designed to improve the profession, often by establishing training or entry examination requirements for a specialty. Professional organizations bring about change by cooperation among members, by professional or patient education, by promoting standards of excellence, and by influencing legislation or policy at many levels.

Professional organizations may be county or state medical societies, state specialty societies (e.g., a society for pathologists or anesthesiologists), national specialty societies, or national professional colleges, such as the American College of Physicians or the American College of Surgeons. A few of our subjects were also involved in national ''cooperative groups'' for developing and implementing various research-oriented patient treatment protocols. One such group was a cooperative oncology group, collaborating in randomized clinical trials for new forms of cancer treatment.

While over half of the twenty-one changes involving physicians and associations related to patient welfare or public policy, the remainder related to the necessary task of maintaining an organization, for example, beginning a new society, being initiated into membership, serving as an officer, and resigning from an association. Patient welfare was effected by work on legislation, by organizing CME programs or teaching in them, by participating in peer review programs, or by initiating new protocols for treatment or immunization.

Peer Review

Peer review is an important activity in medical organizational life. This activity is responsible for programs that adopt and promote high standards for patient care or monitor physician performance. This is accomplished by formally invoking the judgment of other physicians who are peers. At its best, peer review is an activity of the profession itself. According to a recent official statement, such professionally sponsored activity will be strengthened further in the years ahead. Efforts will include reviewing membership lists to identify cases of professional misconduct and incompetence. There also will be activity on the broader aspects of the quality of medical care.

Reviewing past efforts, "physicians and their professional organizations have established a variety of mechanisms to protect the quality of the care of patients . . . the leading clinical and educational journals in medicine [are] published by physician organizations . . . " Furthermore, "[Most] physicians belong to at least one professional organization that has as its principle focus quality assurance, risk management, impaired physician programs or continuing medical education programs" (AMA Board of Trustees 1986). Direct peer review activity or resulting changes were identified in three of the changes relating to organizations. Evidence of the effect of organized peer review also was identified clearly in three cases in the remainder of the chapter; two in hospital groups, one in a partnership. Generally, but not uniformly, physicians were enthusiastic about their professional organizations and described their activities with pride.

CHANGES

Approximately one-quarter of all changes were small, simple accommodations. Half of these were caused by the needs of organizations. Indeed, when change was directed toward the needs of these organizations, accommodation was the most common type of change made. Occasionally, physicians who made these changes reported that they had accumulated the necessary knowledge and skills over many years of participation as members. They noted that the changes did not require much knowledge or skill.

Accommodations caused by associations with partners were infrequent, involving minor changes in practice routines or schedules. Similarly, accommodations associated with relations with informal groups of physicians from hospitals were very minor changes and negatively received.

Adjustments accounted for the majority of changes made by these physicians. Unlike accommodations, these changes were more likely to result from relationships with individuals and partnerships than with hospital groups or formal associations. All changes caused by relationships with other individual physicians were adjustments, and more than two-thirds of changes were driven by relationships with partners. These tended to be changes in methods of diagnosis or care, or less frequently, business or practice arrangements. Four involved an individual partner acting as a consultant who provided information or skills which led to change.

Even though adjustments were less likely to be the products of changes caused by professional organizations, adjustments were common (12 of 21) outcomes when the force for change was relationships to professional organizations. Some of these changes tended to be rather large, such as starting a new journal, organizing and running a CME program, or developing a new patient protocol. Adjustments usually involved learning, when patient care was the issue. This was not as usual when a change related to business procedures or an organizational role. The amount of energy applied to learning was greater when a change was relevant to patient care. Implementing a new drug treatment or a new surgical procedure were typical situations in which the change process was cautiously pursued and validated.

Larger, more complicated changes caused by relationships with others in the profession were rare but dramatic. For example, a urologist, who became disenchanted with his practice group, resigned and set up practice in another town. Such changes required large, complex learning strategies. Overall, physicians who made changes because of their relationships with others in the profession learned as part of the change process. Learning most often was directed toward solving specific, well-defined problems rather than toward acquiring a more basic and general understanding. It often depended on informal resources that were readily available, rather than formal structured resources such as specific courses or seminars. Most often, resources were structured to facilitate thought rather than direct experience.

In more than one-fourth of the changes, CME could be seen to play a role. Almost every conceivable variation of CME was apparent. The educational process might have its origin in formal conferences or meetings, or in publications prepared by national societies. However, its effect also might have appeared in highly informal settings, such as a conversation between two physicians, one of whom had attended a formal meeting, or in a meeting organized within a partnership, for which no formal CME credit was sought. Participation ranged from attending conferences or meetings, to planning them. Nearly all the changes in behavior attributed to CME were in clinical practice (16 of 19 cases). Almost

Table 9.1
Type of Change According to Sources of Pressure for Change

	TYPES					
	Individual	*Covert Peer Pressure*	*Partner*	*Informal Hospital Group*	*Professional Organization*	*Total*
Accomo-dation	0	0	3	5	8	16
Adjust-ment	12	2	11	8	13	45
Redirect-tion	0	1	1	1	0	3
Transfor-mation	0	1	1	0	1	2
Total	12	3	16	14	22	66

always, CME was only one element in a complex of learning activities leading to change.

SUMMARY AND IMPLICATIONS

In this chapter, sixty-six changes were studied in which the driving force for change was how one physician related to another physician or a group of physicians. (See Table 9.1.) Approximately one-fourth of the changes came from relationships with another physician. Three-fourths were changes relating to groups. One-fifth (14 of 66) described activity with a partnership, one-fifth described activities of informal hospital groups, and one-third (21 of 66) were in relation to professional medical organizations.

A key to understanding change driven by relationships among individual physicians is the role of the consultant. A consultation, whether formal or informal, was always associated with changes in patient management; it was almost always an adjustment (there was one exception); and the patient was always at the center of the change process. That is to say, patients caused these relationships and provided occasions for orderly exchanges of views. Consultants play an important role in medicine. They expand the available resources by providing a more explainable armamentarium. They increase the range of professional services available to the referring physician. Consultants also play an ongoing role as their colleagues' teachers.

Physicians may use consultants for primary learning more often than they realize. According to Covell, Uman, and Manning (1985) physicians described themselves as turning to the literature to answer sixty percent of their patient care questions, although they could only be observed to answer about twenty-five percent of their questions in this way. Conversely, they reported using other physicians or health professionals relatively, for thirty-two percent of their answers, whereas the real proportion was fifty-three percent.

Any effort to enhance learning to improve patient care should include close attention to the consultant's role. A special case, the role of mentor, is less common but potentially very powerful. Consultants in medicine are a species of "educational influential" as characterized by Morris (1976). Educational influentials are distinctive in four types of ability: Communications, function, performance, and personal attributes. Training such influentials to educate proves to be an effective method of CME (Stross et al. 1983).

The consultant function also has important implications for educators. If CME planners remain aware of the potentially powerful role that conference-goers, including primary care physicians, play in conveying new information to their colleagues, there could be several improvements in conference design. Well-organized written materials would appear more frequently as adjuncts to CME conferences, and would enhance the role of CME participants as consultant-educators. Perhaps instruction on "what and how to tell the doctors back home" could be attractive additions to some conferences.

The referral process is also an area in which learning takes place. As noted in Shortell's study (1972), "An overlooked feature of the referral process is the important education function that it can perform. Not only does it serve to educate physicians about each other's abilities, but it also establishes regular channels of communication through which he can obtain information about new types of diagnostic and therapeutic techniques." Shortell found that forty-four percent of internists with a subspecialty, and twenty-nine percent of general internists reported frequently learning something from the referral of patients, and the totals were much higher (75 and 78 percent respectively) when those who "at least occasionally learned something" were included.

Accommodations are most common among organizations. They also are found in partnerships and informal groups, but they did not result from relationships among individuals. Accommodations in organizations are related to tasks commonly undertaken for the good of the organization. Absence of accommodations among individuals is explained by the fact that all doctor-to-doctor contacts in this chapter were consultant-driven changes in patient treatment.

Adjustment changes, wherever they occurred, tended to be related to patient care. Physicians described intentional learning activity in three-fourths of cases leading to adjustment changes.

From their own descriptions of the ways they used CME, physicians in practice seemed to be adaptable, flexible, and capable of designing their own learning programs. Whether pursued for formal credit or not, self-designed programs were a useful option for many.

Of the changes observed in relation to professional organizations, half were essentially less relevant to patient care. They represented bureaucratic or organizational events, such as joining, taking office, and so on. The other half included cases of improving patient services or patient education, by using the services and resources of professional organizations, developing and producing CME programs for the organization, or working to bring about change as a public service of the organizations (e.g., lobbying for mandatory seat belt legislation). Policymakers already understand the complexity and power of professional organizations to effect change. It is unlikely that intended changes in policy of interest to these organizations can be carried out effectively without assessing their positions for or against such changes.

The rich networks of professional relationships serve as elaborate systems reviewing the quality of patient care. The best safeguard for patients in a teaching hospital well may be that physicians practice transparently, in a "goldfish bowl," as it were (Knowles 1963). This same fact makes it difficult, in many cases, to assess clearly the impact of a single physician on outcomes of medical care—the more so, in critical illnesses when many specialists are in attendance.

Physicians work together, not in isolation, as they learn and change. Sometimes, in consulting relationships, there is reciprocity of teaching and learning. Both formal and informal organizations serve to maintain stability of medical practice, but also to induce change. Educators, policymakers, and physicians themselves, not to mention patients and the public, will be served well by an increasing understanding of the importance and the utility of these relationships as forces for change.

REFERENCES

American Medical Association, Board of Trustees. Initiative on quality of medical care and professional self regulation. Report QQ, adopted by House of Delegates, June 15–19, 1986. *Journal of the American Medical Association* 256(8):1036–7, August 22–29, 1986.

Covell, D. G., G. C. Uman, and P. R. Manning. 1985. Information needs in office practice: Are they being met? *Annals of Internal Medicine* 103:596–599.

Knowles, J. H. 1963. The balance of biology of the teaching hospital. *New England Journal of Medicine* 269:401–406, 450–455.

Levinson, D. J., et al. 1978. *The seasons of a man's life.* New York: Alfred A. Knopf.

Morris, W. 1976. The information influential physician: The knowledge flow process among medical practitioners. Ph.D. diss. Ann Arbor: University of Michigan.

Shortell, S. M. 1972. *A model of physician referral behavior: A test of exchange theory in medical practice*. Research Series 31. Chicago: Center for Health Administration Studies, University of Chicago.

Stross, J. K., et al. 1983. Continuing education in pulmonary disease for primary-care physicians. *American Review of Respiratory Diseases* 127:739–746.

10

Regulations

Paul E. Mazmanian
and Peter O. Fried

It's the government. They've become intrusive. They have encroached on my relationship with patients. They want to cut costs, so they try to tell me how to practice medicine. If I don't follow their guidelines, the hospital does not get reimbursed, and I've got problems with my colleagues and the hospital administration. If I follow their guidelines, sometimes I have to send patients home before I want to. Patients think I ought to make them better and they expect perfect results, so my medical malpractice insurance premium has tripled over the past four years. I've got to practice medicine in ways I'm not used to just to maintain enough revenue to cover the increase in medical liability premiums and to maintain my income. It's a battle. The fun has been taken out of medicine.

I attended a few programs put on by the hospital when DRGs were first imposed. I can tell you this, the paperwork is incredible. The DRG programs teach you how to cover yourself and the hospital by charting and categorizing. The insurance company sponsored a medical malpractice seminar to teach us to document everything. With all the time I spend writing and documenting every move I make, it's a wonder I get to see patients. The medical school has not been helpful in either of these areas. I'm not sure that they should be. Other than those malpractice and DRG programs, most of the information I get in these areas is from medical colleagues who have experience, or from attorneys and accountants when I pay them.

For several years, personal healthcare expenditures in Canada and the United States have hovered around nine and eleven percent respectively of each country's gross national product (Fuchs 1988). Healthcare expenditures of such great proportion have required regulation. This chapter studies physicians' responses to the regulations intended to assure responsible administration of funds, equitable distribution of high-quality healthcare, and protection for the healthcare consumer. The responses are from physicians who have changed the way they feel about practicing medicine because of being regulated. They feel caught between the drive to cut medical costs and the need to follow their best clinical judgements. They change the way they practice medicine to protect themselves from being sued by patients and because of involvement in peer review systems and quality assurance programs. Nearly half of these changes required no new learning. Physicians simply reflected upon earlier experiences, accepted being regulated as part of professional practice, and adjusted to the rules. The disturbing part is that many of the changes involve emotional responses that tend to signal a profession in distress. Physicians are troubled by needing to make clinical decisions that are heavily influenced by the imposition of non-clinical rules and regulations—rules and regulations that have largely been ignored by the curriculum during clinical training and continue to be ignored by medical schools in continuing education offerings.

FORCES AND CHANGES

For this chapter, regulation is interpreted in a broad sense and includes the following categories: Regulations associated with hospital reimbursement and payment for services, laws as related to medical professional liability, and policies implemented to help assure the public health. Use of these categories enables comparisons and contrasts among and between regulations, changes, and learning.

Hospital Reimbursement and Payment for Services

I have changed the way I evaluate certain Medicare patients, particularly those who have a coin lesion of the lung. The cause of the change was that the clinic received the published list from Medicare of what would and would not be covered for payment. The list stated that bronchoscopies should be performed on an outpatient basis to be assured of coverage by Medicare.

I suspected that performing a bronchoscopy on an outpatient basis could be acceptable except for the case when a patient has a coin lesion, but I needed to be able to back up the contention. I did a literature search and then I tried to affect the Medicare policy by writing to the state organization that is in charge of Medicare. I made a trip to the Capitol to talk to a secretary of the organization, and I wrote a letter arguing against the new policy.

I contacted other major clinics to get ideas about how they have handled the same situation. I did review a triage concept that had been developed several years ago at a medical school, but I did not think it would be helpful in this situation.

Given the time I spent on the literature search and in traveling to the Capitol, as well as in our committee meetings discussing the issue and trying to reach a resolution, I would say I have spent about twenty hours. Probably the most important resources have been the clinic library and contact with other physicians at other clinics.

Regulations associated with reimbursement resulted in thirty-one changes. Specific reasons for change included: (1) the presence of new systems for hospital reimbursement, (2) the development of alternative healthcare delivery systems that involved prospective payment of physicians, and (3) the perceived intrusion of government through regulation of payment. Most of the changes involved negative feelings about these pressures to change. The introduction of diagnostic related groups (DRGs), fee freezes for American physicians, and prospective payment plans, brought about reticence and skepticism, but many of the very same physicians who complained about being compelled to change also expressed concern over rising healthcare costs. They indicated both an understanding of the need to reduce costs, and a frustration with actual cost-cutting measures that may endanger the welfare of patients and increase their risks of professional liability.

Changes in feelings were frequent, usually for the worse, even when simple compliance with rules was reported by interviewees (approximately one-third in this subset were accommodations). Although two physicians reported feeling grateful for the development of a prospective payment system that provided an opportunity to practice in an HMO, nearly all the other (24 of 29) changes made in response to reimbursement regulations were accompanied by negative feelings or descriptions of anxiety. Consternation at the amount of administrative time spent acquiring reimbursement for professional services was typical, as was discontent with prospective payment. Many felt anxiety growing from the need to comply with cost containment measures and, simultaneously, reduce the risks of medical liability. They were anxious about loss of control over the physician-patient relationship, stemming from possible liability associated with actions they may or may not take, based on the current form of reimbursement.

Adjustments in practice management or practice procedures prevailed (19 cases) when reimbursement was an issue. Some physicians (7 of 19) implemented changes in office management, such as increasing or decreasing office hours, automating patient billing, billing patients directly instead of through hospitals, and increasing office efficiency. About half (10 of 19) of the physicians changed one or more procedures from in-patient to out-patient services. Each change was instigated by a DRG requirement. In half of the instances of change to out-patient services, physicians indicated concern regarding the wisdom of reduced in-patient care for specific disorders. Some physicians said they now refer more patients to other specialists, preferring to take less responsibility for the patient's care. One physician said he was seeing more patients as a consultant. Another, a medical school faculty member, said he now sees more patients who earlier would have been seen by residents, in order to protect his income.

The most dramatic response to the imposition of DRGs involved a physician who became angered about the system for payment of physicians, doubled his office hours, added office equipment, and attempted to provide better service to private patients than to publicly-supported patients. He did all of these things hoping to compensate for reduced income associated with "a physician's rate freeze." In contrast, two physicians reacted with more global responses, assuming professional leadership roles, and trying to move organized medicine toward abolition of those laws and regulations that they perceived to be negative influences.

Medical Professional Liability: The Law

In the past year, I stopped "washing ears." I must have washed thousands of them, but this year I had a 74 year old man who experienced pain. I looked and the cerumen was still there, but I thought there might be a perforation. A specialist confirmed my diagnosis. I haven't been sued, but I decided to quit. Let's face it. For washing an ear, I get five dollars. The added premium to cover liability is $3,000. I would need to wash six hundred ears a year to cover the premium. The specialist gets thirty or forty dollars. Let him do it.

I talked with my insurance agent. It did not take long to learn that, for me, the premium did not justify the occasion to treat the case. It is simply economics. I worry a lot more about malpractice, and threat of malpractice, than I used to. I have read enough about it, and I think it's a dark cloud that looms over the practice of medicine. It affects my day-to-day practice, and I'm certain it affects the day-to-day practice of my colleagues. You worry about getting a bad result. You begin to see patients as potential litigants. I feel as if I screen my patients early on to see if they are the type that might be likely to sue.

The rising tide of medical malpractice suits and rapidly increasing rates for medical professional liability insurance brought widespread concern to the medical community. Twenty-six changes resulted from the subset of forces seen as laws affecting professional liability. In another ten cases, although the changes were primarily because of reimbursement regulations, medical liability played a secondary but important role.

There were three reasons for change associated with professional liability: (1) current or past experience in claim resolution, (2) a colleague's involvement in the resolution of a claim, and (3) physicians' perceptions that they might be sued. Accommodations to the professional liability problem (9 of 26 changes in this subset of forces) included reducing the number of hours spent in practice, dampening enthusiasm for the practice of medicine, bringing oneself up to date in one's specialty, adapting psychologically to a professional life that includes the threat of litigation, and increasing general awareness of the threat of professional liability. A few physicians were actively considering early retirement because of the pressures of a litigious physician-patient relationship. One practiced in a small community where, historically, physicians have been difficult to recruit.

In attempts to reduce the likelihood of being sued, about half of the physicians (12 of 26) reported taking defensive measures. Such measures included providing information about several types of treatment (e.g., birth control) and allowing the patient to choose from the alternatives, rather than recommending an approach. Defensive medicine also included the increased use of tests, not so much to add veracity to clinical judgment, but rather to minimize the physicians' vulnerability to claims of medical malpractice. A few physicians screened patients from their practices based on high-risk clinical problems, or because they were viewed by the physician as patients likely to file a malpractice claim. Others reported keeping more complete and accurate patient records, securing more detailed informed consent, and increasing their awareness of the importance of clear communication with patients. In contrast to these adjustments, a 66-year-old physician responded to the experience of being sued by reducing his obstetrics/gynecology practice and becoming semiretired, a redirection of his career.

Most of the physicians (20 of 26) who indicated changes caused by liability issues suggested that the situation was due to patients' unreasonable expectations about the outcome of medical treatment, the growing number of attorneys looking for potential liability cases, the reluctance of patients to accept responsibility for the outcomes of their illnesses, and an increasingly litigious society.

Quality Assurance, Peer Review, and the Government: Health Policy

It happened because I was asked to participate in the peer review system. The system calls for two colleagues to review at random the medical records and practices of physicians in practice. I was asked to attend a one-day conference to prepare me as a reviewer. During the conference I was presented with examples of adequate and inadequate records, and we discussed the many problems that can arise from inadequate records. Since then, and having participated in at least twenty visits to other physicians' offices, I have instituted a new recordkeeping system that I believe has helped to improve the quality of care by providing me with information on dosages of drugs, their duration, specific investigative techniques, including results and information for a much more thorough assessment of the patient. I have also recommended to hospital administration that a similar hospital-wide information system could enable us to strengthen some of the weaknesses identified during our last accreditation visit.

Health policy provides governing principles to support prudent management of resources allocated to help assure the public's health. Reported as peer review, quality assurance, occupational safety, hospital accreditation, and other systems of standards and reviews, the subset of regulations discussed in this section includes those arising from the implementation of health policy. Health policy caused fewer changes (16 of 73) than other forms of regulations. The primary reasons for change cited by physicians were the desire to gain or maintain practice privileges, and the need to interpret the law to help assure patient or public safety.

One of every four changes caused by health policies was characterized by physicians acknowledging, implementing, or complying with new written standards. Half of these changes involved physicians whose practices were based in federal or state institutions and included compliance with new admission or discharge criteria. The need to comply with Joint Commission on Accreditation of Healthcare Organizations (JCAHO) standards was a motivating force leading one physician to accept an administrative assignment to help assure that his hospital would meet those standards. Another change involved a private practitioner, a 67-year-old anesthesiologist, who indicated that medicine had suffered too much government encroachment. "If I were younger," he said, "I'd consider something else."

Most of the changes (10 of 16) resulting from health policy were adjustments. Nearly half of these involved peer review systems such as ethics panels, routine audits of hospital charts for quality assurance, or professional review organizations (PROs)—federally sponsored groups in the United States—assigned to monitor records in an effort to help assure that cost effective care, meeting proscribed minimal standards, is provided through the Medicare system. Three of the four physicians attributing changes to peer review had been subjects of review. Although two reported changes in methods of patient care to satisfy criteria, one developed a strategy for satisfying his PRO without changing methods of patient care. The fourth physician had served as a peer reviewer and had changed her patient record keeping habits as a result. Additionally, she was encouraging adoption of a new records system for the hospital, because of what she learned during her experience as a reviewer.

Other adjustments included a medical school faculty member who refocused his research interests and found new practice opportunities due to threatened cuts in federal funding; and a practitioner who actively prepared for his retirement, as required by corporate rules derived from mandatory retirement age legislation. Two physicians, specializing in occupational medicine, created programs to implement laws designed to protect pregnant women in the workplace and disabled workers in job assignments. One military physician took charge of an effort to reformulate credentialing and quality assurance requirements, anticipating budget reductions and the need to meet JCAHO standards.

A physician whose practice had been the object of peer review reported a major redirection of his career by resigning his administrative position within the hospital, reducing the time spent on patient care, and increasing his efforts to influence congressmen and other policymakers regarding the weaknesses of the Medicare system. Another complex change occurred when a physician dropped his private consulting practice at a state hospital, accepted a full-time faculty position funded by the Veterans Administration (whose regulations prohibited him from continuing to see private patients), and initiated planning for a consulting service that would provide experience for resident physicians, and enable the state hospital to meet JCAHO requirements for an external quality of care monitor.

LEARNING

Nearly half of the changes caused by regulation were made without physicians engaging in reported new learning activities (34 of 73). This compared with less than one-third of the changes for the overall study. When learning was involved in changes caused by being regulated, it most often was associated with adjustments resulting from medical professional liability (10 of 15 changes) and health policies (8 of 10 changes). Adjustments due to reimbursement regulations were as likely as not (9 of 19) to involve learning. The lower prevalence of learning in changes driven by regulations seemed to be related to the small and simple nature of changes, and negative attitudes toward regulations.

Although most physicians indicated that medical schools were not helpful in changes associated with regulations, many indicated that schools could be. They said they would prefer to have medical schools be responsible for programs currently presented by hospitals, accounting firms, attorneys, insurance companies, and government agencies.

Reimbursement

Regulations for reimbursement occasionally caused accommodations. Usually, these involved assimilation of information from journals, discussion with hospital administrators, and attendance at national specialty or professional society meetings (6 of 11). Similarly, only nine of the nineteen adjustments associated with reimbursement involved new learning. When learning was part of these incremental changes in patient care, it usually included informal discussions with colleagues. When the changes involved office management, they were more likely to include learning from formal sources, usually in sessions conducted by people less directly involved in patient care, such as ethicists, hospital administrative staff, or computer software consultants. The most extended learning project involved planned educational programs, journal reading, and other self-instruction, over a period of three years, to facilitate the introduction of computers into the office system.

Medical Professional Liability

When an accommodation to the law was the outcome, there was usually no reported new learning (7 of 9 changes) associated with the change. Awareness and sensitivity to professional liability as a threat, as well as anger or concern over the increasing rate of malpractice claims and the size of awards against physicians, were often the outcomes of pressure from the laws governing professional liability. Information was acquired through journals, colleagues, the lay press, or other readily available sources. Many of the same information sources were utilized when adjustments such as ordering more tests, more cautious recordkeeping, and screening of patients were made. However, these physicians also sought consultations from insurance representatives and attorneys. Methods and resources for learning included private consultations, educational conferences, pamphlets, newsletters, and audiotapes. Physicians in the midst of medical malpractice suits and involved in large complex changes (redirection and transformation) also utilized reviews of patient records, scientific and legal accounts of similar cases, reviews of testimony taken during interrogatories, and consultations with defense attorneys.

Physicians involved in, or concerned about malpractice litigation, perceived the forces of liability as a threat to the profession. They used information to define the problem and to generate workable alternatives to solve problems associated with medical professional liability. Others saw professional liability as something that needed to be understood in conceptual terms. There was an expectation among the latter group that acquiring information from bona fide written sources and medical colleagues would provide clear methods for defensive practices that would protect them from malpractice claims. In contrast, the physicians involved in complex career changes believed the allegations brought against them stemmed not from their wrong doing but from some other motivation driving the patient to use the legal system.

Health Policy

As with liability concerns, accommodations caused by health policies typically required no new learning (3 of 4). All four, however, included changes in orientation and a general dissatisfaction toward compliance with new or altered policies (see Table 10.1). In contrast to the redirection and transformation changes caused by concerns over professional liability, no new learning was described for either of the redirections caused by health policy. Physicians changed career roles, in part, because they sensed oppressive limitations resulting from health policy.

CONCLUSIONS, DISCUSSION, AND IMPLICATIONS

1. *Three subsets of regulations were evident as forces for change.*

Regulations associated with hospital reimbursement and physician payment, the laws governing medical professional liability, and health policy designed to help assure the public safety and a high standard of care, were all forces for change. The first subset of regulations is aimed at medical cost containment. The second subset is intended to guarantee that patients can find justice and, ultimately, secure compensation if injured because of a physician's actions or lack of care. The third is meant both to enfranchise groups that implement medical quality assurance and to direct individuals authorized to interpret the laws protecting citizens. The presence of all these rules for regulating practice demon-

Table 10.1
Component Forces and Learning Associated With Types of Change

Component Forces & Learning	Types of Change			
	Accomo-dation	Adjust-ment	Redirec-tion	Transfor-mation
Reimbursement Regulations				
Learning	6 (38%)	9 (56%)	1 (6%)	0
No New Learning	5 (33%)	10 (67%)	0	0
Medical Professional Liability				
Learning	21 (14%)	10 (71%)	1 (7%)	1 (7%)
No New Learning	7 (58%)	5 (42%)	0	0
Health Care Policy				
Learning	1 (11%)	8 (89%)	0	0
No New Learning	3 (43%)	2 (29%)	2 (29%)	0
TOTALS Learning	9 (23%)	27 (69%)	2 (5%)	1 (3%)
No New Learning	15 (44%)	17 (50%)	2 (6%)	0
Grand Totals	24	44	4	1

strates that society has chosen to express its concerns over the quality and price of medical care, in part, through the regulation of medical practices and the systems that support it.

Obtaining reimbursement for services was reported frequently to be burdensome, disconcerting, and time-consuming, resulting in less time for patient care. Despite the widespread reports of deep-seated concern, however, there were no reported instances of physicians leaving professional practice because of paperwork involved with Medicare/Medicaid and DRGs, or their associated fee freezes. It generally was understood by physicians that healthcare costs must be controlled, however, new systems were viewed with anxiety and caution by most physicians.

2. *Change in response to regulations was usually small, involving psychological repositioning or limited adjustment in practice.*

The three subsets of regulations did not differ from one another in terms of their consequences. In general, they led to a disproportionate number of willing or unwilling small, simple changes. One in every three changes associated with regulations was an accommodation, compared with one in five for the overall study. About one in every twenty changes caused by regulations was large and complex, compared with one in every eight for all changes in the study.

Regulation proved to be effective in changing physician behavior, but it also proved to be a powerful source of antagonism, fostering ill will among physicians, as well as between physicians and patients, administrators, and policymakers. The inevitable clash of a fiercely independent profession and the forces that try to control it is apparent. Every practicing physician now is compelled to maintain familiarity with ever-changing regulations spewing from government and private agencies; and changes resulting from those regulations involve areas in which physicians are largely untrained, such as medical economics, practice management, the law, and development of health policies. Despite the physician's limited training in these areas, the financial and professional viability of the physician's practice, as well as the success of the hospital or other healthcare organization, are directly related to the physician's interpretation and compliance with these new regulations.

Change in areas that require new expertise also bred anxiety. Many felt torn by the belief that, for society, the value of cost containment has become more important than highest quality medical care and the responsibility to help patients feel better. Physicians understandably disagreed with these priorities because they traditionally have idealized the ethic of duty to their patients. They did not recognize compliance with or minor adjustment to cost containment regulations as change. Rather, it often was seen as integral to their role as a healthcare provider. The conflict of regulations, particularly cost containment and professional liability, sparked considerable bravado, anger, and expressions of woe from these physicians, who saw themselves at the center of conflict. Even though powerful, mounting pressure was indeed a source of stress, the changes they made were mostly limited in scope, depth, and alternately, in dedication.

3. *Physicians are angry, frustrated and resistant to change caused by regulations.*

Many physicians expressed the belief that their interests are not being served by those in political and economic control of the healthcare system. A few believe that to oppose those responsible for these "fundamental changes in healthcare," they must adopt a unified strategy and amass political and economic power enough to countermand the pressure for change. Most physicians in this study reported compliance with regulations and the law, as well as limited new learning associated with that compliance, but at the same time, expressed substantial dissatisfaction with the overall system of regulating healthcare.

Regulation seems to divide the medical community. Physicians argue between themselves over "how" or "if" they should participate in professional review organizations. They disagree among and between specialties whether surgical procedures should be reimbursed at higher rates than nonsurgical care. They struggle to decide whether to associate with healthcare corporations as employees, contractors, or limited partners, or to compete by organizing their own businesses. Their opinions are divided by their beliefs and the values they assign to each organizational relationship.

Some of the dissatisfaction with regulation may be related to the gap between physicians' expectations of what the physician/patient relationship ought to be and what it has become. Physicians, in large measure, are defined by their professional training, commitment to patient care, and medical practice. Personal, professional, and financial well-being are interrelated, determined in part by the physicians' success as promoters of healing and by the exercise of privileges associated with practice in a premier profession. Many physicians view recent changes in reimbursement systems, the law, and efforts at quality assurance as assaults upon the sanctity of the physician/patient relationship, and as concerted attacks on the integrity of the medical profession, as well as on the stability and standard of living that have attended the practice of modern medicine. The adjustments that physicians make in being regulated most often are minimal responses intended to reduce the effects of the regulations and to preserve their personal, professional, and financial well-being. Physicians have been forced to integrate ways of changing into their practices and their lives without having had the benefit of participation in development of these regulations. Moreover they have not had the benefit of education designed to help them respond to regulations.

4. *Regulations as a force for change do not generate new learning.*

About half the changes caused by each subset of regulations required no new learning. This compared with less than one-third for the overall study. Nearly two of every three accommodations required no new learning. Nearly four of every ten adjustments required no new learning compared with one of ten for the study.

The low incidence of reported new learning associated with the high ratio of smaller changes depicts the effects of resistance to change by physicians, who perceive a loss of privileges and power over their personal and professional lives. Chin and Benne (1976) explain:

Some of the difficulty with the use of political institutions to effect changes arises from an overestimation by change agents (those stimulating, proposing or implementing the change) of the capability of political action to effect changes in practice. When the law is passed, the administrative ruling announced, or the judicial decision handed down legitimizing some new policy or program or illegitimizing some traditional practice, change agents who have worked hard for the law, ruling, or decision frequently assume that the desired change has been made.

Actually all that has been done is to bring the force of legitimacy behind some envisioned change. The processes of re-education of persons who are to conduct themselves in new ways still have to be carried out.

As the reports of change in this chapter show, the education of physicians to changes in law, economics, and health policy has been uncoordinated and largely ignored by medical schools. Physicians have been left to their own devices in educating themselves through consultation with attorneys, administrators, sales representatives, and others who usually are not directly involved in patient care, or they must become involved in solving an immediate problem, requiring a crash review of administrative material and patient records, followed by on-the-job experience. Many physicians feel unprepared, embattled, and frustrated by this recurring scenario. Such self-directed learning is not unusual among the professional classes. Rather, it has become the norm (Tough 1978).

Brookfield (1984) suggests that most professionals are only partially aware of their roles as self-directed learners, having had no explicit preparation in that regard. Building on Schon's (1987) theory of reflective action and learning, Nowlen (1988, 204) recently wrote:

The most commonly self-directed learning is a seamless, reflective conversation of the professional with the practice situation. It is so much a piece of each professional act that it is virtually impossible to distinguish action from reflection. The reflective act of practice is the elemental, atomic structure of self-directed learning in the professions.

Schon (1987) explains that such learning is observable in the skillful execution of performance, and that professionals are characteristically unable to make the process verbally explicit.

Since the present study focused only on new learning as part of the process of changing, it is likely that physicians did not recognize their considerations of previous experiences as reflective, self-directed learning. Such description would have required reference to, or construction of, concepts similar to those asserted by Brookfield, Nowlen, and Schon, concepts with which physicians are generally unfamiliar.

Discussion

To better understand change caused by regulation, it seems important to consider the recent reorganization of healthcare in the United States and the social value placed on healthcare in Canada. The federal government is the largest purveyor of health insurance in the United States, and as such, has been largely responsible for converting the fundamental, retrospective fee-for-services system of medical care to one involving prospective payment and standardized fee schedules. Much of the premium once placed on increased medical services delivered to a patient has changed to an economic incentive for fewer medical services provided to more patients. The pivotal point in this drive toward cost containment occurred in 1983, with freezes on Medicare fee schedules for physicians, and the introduction of DRGs (a system of reimbursement that presets payment to hospitals based on diagnostically-related groups of patients, illnesses, and average length of stay). The drive to reduce costs also provided fertile ground for the development of HMOs, with the number of HMO patients swelling to more than eighteen million in 1985, from seven million in 1978 (Tarlov 1986). In addition, the past few years have seen extensive legal activity concerning malpractice and antitrust suits in medicine (Curran 1989). Such sweeping change has required personal and professional reorientation of practitioners' responsibilities to their patients, the hospital, the medical profession, and ultimately to themselves.

Virtually all of Canada's 25.5 million citizens receive care through a publicly financed healthcare system. The system was designed to protect Canadians from the economic consequences of illness. It was also designed to limit the government's financial commitment and to preserve the autonomy of its private physicians. The relative independence of Canada's hospitals also was to be assured.

In his review of the Canadian healthcare system, Iglehart (1986) finds that major budget deficits of the Canadian government have caused the healthcare system to strain under the pressures of regular use and ready access to care for all. Provinces are receiving less in federal support for their health insurance plans, and they are being forced to increase their own fundings of the plans or cut back current expenditures. Physicians' fee schedules are structured so that increases in billings require additional time in practice. The number of hours in a day, then, constrains the expansion of physicians' billings. Physicians have been asked to stop billing patients at rates above government-approved payment levels, an action seen by many as a sharp blow to professionalism in medicine.

The stories of change reported in this chapter indicate that learning and change caused by being regulated are limited, but emotions and resistance run high. Physicians, educators, and policymakers all have an interest in assuring that change is promoted and implemented in an efficient manner. The implications for such practice need to be examined.

Two classic works on planned change and learning shed some light on the change process and the need to educate for change. Regulations may be seen as methods of diffusing planned innovations (ideas and practices) in healthcare. Rogers (1983) describes the diffusion of innovations as ideas, practices, or objects that are perceived as new by an individual who may adopt the innovations. Rogers contends that so far as human behavior is concerned, whether or not an idea is "objectively" new, as measured by the lapse of time since its first use or discovery, is inconsequential. If the idea seems new to an individual, it is an innovation. The success of diffusion of innovations is dependent upon several characteristics:

1. *Relative advantage* is the degree to which an innovation is perceived as better than the idea it supercedes.
2. *Compatibility* is the degree to which an innovation is perceived as being consistent with the existing values, past experiences, and needs of potential adopters.
3. *Complexity* is the degree to which an innovation is perceived as difficult to understand and use.
4. *Trialability* is the degree to which an innovation may be experimented with on a limited basis.
5. *Observability* is the degree to which the results of an innovation are visible to others. (Rogers, 1983, pp. 223–234).

Diffusion theory allows one to predict changes in practice according to the extent to which innovations are perceived as having greater relative advantage, compatibility, trialability, observability, and less complexity.

Chin and Benne (1976) identify three types of strategies for changing: Empirical-rational, normative-reeducative, and power coercive. Each change strategy has limitations:

1. *Empirical-rational* approaches are limited in that the person proposing the change must first show the person or group (assumed to be rational and moved by self-interest) that there is benefit to changing. Scientific investigation and research represent the chief ways of extending knowledge and reducing the limitations of ignorance.
2. With *normative-reeducative* strategies, patterns of action and practice must be supported by sociocultural norms, involving attitude and value systems of individuals and groups. Change occurs only as the persons associated are brought to change their normative orientations involving changes in attitudes, values, skills, and significant relationships—not just changes in knowledge, information, or intellectual rationales for action and practice.
3. Political and economic sanctions are emphasized in the exercise of *power-coercive* strategies. Knowledge is a less important ingredient. Political and economic power are amassed behind change goals chosen by those who are promoting change. The planners assume that change will not occur without legitimized power driving the change process.

From Chin and Benne, one sees that learning is not essential to change caused by regulations enforced through political and economic sanctions. Resistance to such change is likely to be high, and change is likely to be as small and simple as possible.

Regulations are attempts to implement change. If we want physicians to understand change and the reasons for it, the current strategy for planned change should be reconsidered. If the plan is to change the ways people act toward one another or the ways they interrelate with new technologies, the processes of introducing such changes must be based on behavioral knowledge of change. The plan should utilize methods for change that are based on such knowledge. Physician participation throughout the planning and implementation of change appears critical to a successful change effort.

Most physicians currently in practice were trained with a set of expectations regarding the sanctity of the physician-patient relationship, remuneration for services, responsibilities of office management, and personal as well as social role expectations of medical professionals. For fifty years or more, those expectations have remained fundamentally unchanged, but during a comparatively short period of time, the stability and promise of a career in medicine have been essentially reformed. Policymakers must provide a sense of understanding responsive to the threatened stability of practicing physicians.

Policymakers must find meaningful roles for physicians in the development and implementation of programs that support the delivery of high-quality healthcare as well as ready access to healthcare. They must gather data for analysis of patient care outcomes to allow meaningful correlations and comparisons among and between systems for the delivery of healthcare. Physicians and policymakers should work with medical educators to assure that the medical school curriculum is one that is responsive to changes in a closely regulated healthcare environment.

Physicians have been trained to provide the highest quality care available and to treat the physician-patient relationship as sacred. As cost containment and medical professional liability have influenced the physician-patient relationship, and as certain strategies have been designed to regulate directly the physician-patient relationship, professional and personal conflict have resulted. Medical educators must be sensitive to changes impinging on the clinical environment. They should prepare physicians to consider the physician-patient relationship in organizational and economic terms as well as in an individual clinical sense. Ethical decisions must be made explicit. Data on the outcome and quality of care should be studied, and the curriculum should be altered to include selected non-clinical information throughout the continuum of medical education.

Although medical schools have not been helpful in learning associated with changes in reimbursement, medical professional liability, and health policy, many physicians rely upon medical schools as trusted sources for continuing education. They have expected medical schools to foster and protect the essential acculturation of young doctors, and to sanction as "valid and reliable" medical breakthroughs for practicing physicians. Throughout undergraduate, graduate, and continuing medical education, the medical curriculum has been inattentive to non-clinical issues, seen as indirectly affecting patient care—issues such as economics, practice management, and professional liability. Medical schools should now complete the contract with physician-learners and with patients. They need to adjust the traditional curriculum to include non-clinical information that enables physicians to adjust to change and participate in the regulatory process. Medical schools must teach physicians critical appraisal skills that will enable them to glean the merits of innovations and pass them along as benefits to their patients. They also must teach physicians to challenge change when that is appropriate.

Many questions remain about changes associated with regulations. How long do small, simple changes made because of regulations endure? What are the most effective ways of recruiting and integrating positive physician involvement in change and learning caused by regulation? What conditions facilitate or promote regulation-induced change in a physician's practice? Can the ability to implement change, or successfully adjust to change, be taught? How are the skills of critical appraisal and effective decision making effectively taught to medical students, medical practitioners, and others involved in the change process? If we want physicians to understand change and the reasons for it, we must educate them to it. Without more attention to the study of change, regulations, and learning, attempts to bring about change by health policymakers, medical educators, and professional organizations are more likely to fail because of predictable resistance to being regulated.

REFERENCES

Brookfield, S. D. 1984. *Adult learners, adult education, and the community.* New York: Teachers College Press.

Chin, R., and K. D. Benne. 1976. General strategies for effecting changes in human systems. In Bennis, W. G., et al. *The planning of change* 3d ed. New York: Holt, Rinehart, and Winston.

Curran, W. J. (1989) Legal immunity for medical peer-review programs. *New England Journal of Medicine* 320:233–235.

Fuchs, V. R. 1988. Perspectives: United States. *Health Affairs* 7(5):25–30.

Iglehart, J. K. 1986. Health policy report: Canada's health care system. *New England Journal of Medicine* 315:778–784.

Nowlen, P. M. 1988. *A new approach to continuing education for business and the professions.* New York: Macmillan.

Rogers, E. M. 1983. *Diffusion of innovations.* 3d ed. New York: The Free Press.

Schon, D. A. 1987. *Educating the reflective practitioner.* San Francisco: Jossey-Bass.

Tarlov, A. R. 1986. HMO growth and physicians. *Health Affairs* 5(1):23–35.

Tough, A. M. 1978. Major learning efforts: Recent research and future directions. *Adult Education* 29(4):250–263.

11
Family and Community

Jacqueline Parochka
and Robert D. Fox

> I've learned that being a doctor, and a parent, and a wife, doesn't always
> go together. Sometimes they conflict and, when they do, something has to
> give. I have friends who have given up their families or who have stopped
> certain parts of their practices to find the time to do what needs to be done.
> What makes it worse is that as you get older, it seems like your practice
> and your family demand more and more. Basically, I have had to adjust my
> practice to avoid being on call, so there's more time to do what I've got to
> do as a spouse and a mother. I can't say that I'm happy about this change,
> but I don't believe I would be happy about making any more changes in
> the way I fulfill my obligations at home. It's been a problem I have had to
> do a lot of thinking about. The hardest part has been finding good information
> that is relevant. I've used everything from journal articles to private dis-
> cussions with friends and neighbors to consider the alternatives and cope
> with the pressure of having what you might call too many jobs. In medical
> school people talked about the pressures of being a doctor, but too often
> you got the feeling that whenever these pressures conflicted with the pressures
> of your other roles, you should just be a doctor. It would help to be better
> prepared to face all the expectations of everyone without feeling a little
> guilty about what you're not doing.

In talking about her struggle to reconcile the demands of parenting and doctoring,
this physician refers to conflicts between her different "roles." Although it is
a cliche, the notion of *roles* as a way of organizing social life has its uses. The
term was borrowed from the theater by the dramaturgical school of sociology,

as exemplified in a work by Goffman (1959). Social situations are interpreted as scenes in a play. The ''scripts'' for these scenes are derived from consensus about how the various participants should behave. To a remarkable degree, people seek to learn and deliver their lines in ways that they believe are appropriate. Part of the force of this metaphor derives from the fact that people do tend to recognize their social attitudes, actions, and responses as being, at least partly, scripted for them. A role may become a source of tension, and therefore of change, when it is altered in a way the actor did not anticipate on first assuming it. And since most people play more than one role, there is always potential for the demands of one to conflict with those of another.

As a rule, each of us assumes one professional role that may or not provide a dominant identity. Parent, spouse, schoolboard member, amateur athlete, or stamp collector—are other roles, centered in family or community, that come with more or less well-defined standards for performance. How well any one of them is filled depends on the actor's ability to read the script (that is, to perceive the expectations attached to the role) and perform accordingly. Failure generates pressure, originating with others or the self, to change.

Quite apart from the ordinary problems of ability (is A smart enough to be a surgeon, agile enough to be an acrobat, or holy enough to be a minister?), roles themselves can generate a sense of failure or pressure to change. The role of physician, for example, comes with a confusing script in contemporary America. A good doctor is expected, on one hand, to have a warm personality, compassionate attitudes, and a humane concern for patients as whole people. But the good doctor should also maintain the highest levels of technical competence, and an encyclopedic knowledge of medicine, one that requires an almost computer-like mentality to acquire and apply. These aspects of the ideal doctor may be seen as incompatible with each other, and may generate a sense of conflict *within* the role itself. Of course, other roles (for example, that of mother) can also be fraught with complexity and contradiction.

Roles are also subject to recasting by social and historical forces—creating the sense that the actor no longer is playing true to type. Medicine may once have been perceived as being among the last professional refuges for individualism and autonomy; and the doctor who entered his or her profession with that concept may have come to believe that the script now calls for a bureaucrat, and consequently feels ill-suited to the performance.

Although the role of physician has sometimes been seen as requiring a monastic dedication, most doctors and most of their patients appear to reject the notion that someone cloistered in the profession, without experiencing the complexities of life in the family or community, is the optimal practitioner. In any case, relatively few people choose such an impoverished repertoire for themselves. But the moment one assumes a second, third, or fourth role in life, the potential for conflict between one role and another is established.

As members of their families and communities, the physicians in our sample were dealing with the pressures of definition, change, and conflict in these "private" areas. We recorded forty-two episodes of change that were driven by expectations arising from roles in the family or community. Marriages dissolved, clinical practices changed, lifestyles were altered, and emotions ranging from guilt to relief were expressed by physicians coping with the requirements of their "other life"—the family and community responsibilities outside medical practice.

Pressures were mainly of two types: New or altered *expectations* for performance in community or family roles, and *conflict* between professional and civic or family obligations. Of the forty-two cases of change we recorded, twenty-six were driven by attempts to meet changing role expectations and sixteen were driven by attempts to resolve conflicting expectations. Among the causes of altered role expectations were new marriages or new obligations within an existing partnership; calls for parental input, ranging from the illness of a young child to the divorce of a grown child; and duties in community organizations, such as a school board, PTA, church, or synagogue. Role conflict was also experienced as a forced choice as to where time would be spent, attention applied, or physical and emotional energies expended—mainly experienced as a conflict between professional and family claims on the physician's resources. But conflict was also perceived as arising from the different nature of emotional, physical, and social demands in the two spheres.

These pressures prompted the doctors to talk about confusion over what they "ought to be doing" and how hard it was to "reconcile their time to their responsibilities." A wide range of responses was evident—among them divorce, reduced size of practice, new babies, and changes in clinical procedures. Many of these changes were described as intended to relieve distress. To find relief from the stress of changing or conflicting roles, the physicians, on the whole, chose one of three tactics: Comply with the script, abandon the role, or redefine it.

Compliance was nearly the universal response to changing role expectations (21 of 26 cases), whereas it characterized just over half of the responses to role conflict (10 of 16 cases). Compliant behaviors included such simple responses as making space for a mother-in-law when she wanted to move in, finding a separate room for a new wife's pets, accepting a deaconship in a church, assuming a committee responsibility in a synagogue, and buying a new house. However, it also entailed more complicated behavior, as in the case of a physician who, because it was his parental duty, formed a private corporation to transport children to school, so that his own child's transportation problems could be solved. Another became fed up with the performance of his child's school and successfully ran for the community's school board.

Some aspect of medical practice also might be altered as part of the compliance tactic. One physician, for example, moved her office setting so that she could go home and be with her newborn baby as often as possible. Others changed work schedules to provide more time to be with family, or relocated to provide opportunity for a professional spouse.

A more drastic type of response, entirely abandoning a role, was less common than compliance. There were six of these, and five were occasioned by role conflict rather than change. Two doctors described divorces: One driven by the heavy role expectations of a particular marriage, and the other based on conflicts between the requirements of a large clinical practice and the responsibilities of marriage. In contrast, two physicians reported abandoning an obstetrics/gynecology practice for a more limited general practice, and another described abandoning a successful walk-in clinic group practice to develop a very limited solo practice closer to home.

In some cases, physicians changed their definitions of roles, rather than their own self-concepts or their own situations. Rather than accept or abandon the requirements of jobs, they changed job descriptions. In all, there were seven such cases. For example, because of her experience with her own child's needs and her apprehensions about the child's medical care, one physician altered the way she practiced medicine. She allotted more time to get acquainted with each child, playing and reading stories to allay the child's fears. Her experience as a mother created a conflict with her prior conception of the way a doctor should perform. She resolved it by redefining how a doctor ought to act. One male physician redefined his role of husband and father after experiencing great conflict between the demands of his medical practice and the needs of his wife for support as she pursued a new career. He now spends more time with his children, fixing their meals, transporting them, and helping them with their daily routines, seeing all this as part of his new definition of what it means to be a good father. A third physician faced with conflicts between his medical practice and his family (conflicts that were taking him toward divorce), dropped his active practice, went into subspecialty training in geriatrics, and relocated to a new city where there were more opportunities for both him and his wife to perform their "new roles" as they had defined them. Although not all redefinitions of role expectations were as dramatic as these, they tended to be larger in scope than other changes, and more likely to occur as a result of changing role expectations than as a result of role conflicts.

The various types of change we have described ranged in magnitude from accommodations to transformations (as the terms are used in this volume), and the extent of change, on this scale, was not clearly correlated with the pattern of response (complaince with, abandonment of, or redefinition of a role). "Compliance," in other words, is not synonymous with "accommodation." For example, the physician who dropped obstetrics and gynecology from his practice, in an effort to comply with family expectations, redirected his professional life (in a fairly large group) in order to comply with the expectations of the parenting role, as he saw them.

In three cases, major changes in viewpoint (transformations) took place, each described as a function of role pressures. In two of these cases, as role expectations changed, the physicians redefined their roles. Major changes in direction, described in five cases, were nearly equally likely to result from role conflicts as from role expectations, and in three of five instances were associated with the abandonment of roles.

LEARNING AND CHANGING

In recounting the ways they changed their family and community lives, the physicians reported that they used learning as a tool only half the time, whereas the rate for all instances of change recorded in this study was closer to two-thirds. It may be that there was no clear way to go about learning that was needed in this context; certainly, educational programs directed to the "other life" of physicians rarely are available. It may also be that the physicians did not view knowledge or skill as necessary, to the extent that compliance with changing family or community roles was the predominant response. Whether change was driven by expectations or conflicts seemed to make no difference in learning behavior. Learning was more likely to be directed toward solving a real-life problem than to generating a better general understanding (13 to 8), was more likely to take the form of contemplation or deliberation than interaction or experience (13 to 8), and was slightly more likely to emphasize formal rather than informal learning resources (11 to 10). Deliberation was more than twice as prevalent in this area as in the total cases of change. These relationships are summarized in Table 11.1.

Women are overrepresented among the physicians reporting change in relation to family and community roles (21 percent, compared with 13 percent of physicians interviewed), hardly a surprise in view of the high levels of stress experienced by female professionals who must perform exceptionally well at several exceptionally demanding roles (Rinke 1981; and Heins 1985). The average age of respondents was 43.3 years, and although faculty physicians constituted approximately twenty percent of all respondents for the study, they were only twelve percent of the respondents reporting pressures from family or community roles as forces for change. Perhaps faculty are protected by a more structured system, with more back-up and more well-defined obligations than are non-faculty physicians.

CONCLUSIONS

Doctors may be particularly vulnerable to conflict between professional and nonprofessional roles, because the professional expectations of doctors are so pervasive, and yet, their status in society also creates an expectation of high-level interaction with family and community. Priorities for action become difficult to set. Whether to spend a little more time with the patients or a little more time with the family, whether to maintain a detached professional demeanor in the face of a family crisis or to be a warm and compassionate friend in the face of a patient's crisis, represent the real-life conflicts implicit in many of these stories of change.

Table 11.1
Forces for Change and Learning Strategies

Learning Strategies		Forces for Change		
		Changing Role Expectations	Role Conflicts	Total
Purpose	Conceptual	5	3	8
	Problem Specific	10	3	13
Method	Deliberative	9	4	13
	Experiential	6	2	8
Resources	Formal	9	2	11
	Informal	6	4	10
No learning		11	10	21
		26	16	42

Women physicians are more likely than men to feel the pressures of role expectations and role conflicts. Typecast in social and emotional roles that emphasize compassion, sensitivity, and emotion, women as physicians find themselves in a system that ostensibly values distance, objectivity, and efficiency (Rinke, 1981). Although many of these ideas about sex role differences are coming to be regarded as outdated, female physicians reported that the conflicts and difficulties wrought by such conflicting expectations are still with them and are a wellspring of distress.

The most common type of role-related change was to comply with the requirements of the various roles. Performance was sometimes significantly adjusted to match expectations or resolve conflicts. Occasionally, abandonment of a role was seen as the only acceptable means of coping. Rather than complying or abandoning their roles, some physicians successfully redefined their conceptions of the roles in order to continue in them.

Role expectations, rather than conflicts, were more common incentives to change. When role conflicts did appear, they were more likely to be occasions of role definition or abandonment than of attempts to comply with the scripts as written. In effect, physicians felt more comfortable adding new duties and responsibilities than retaining duties and responsibilities that appeared inconsistent with one another. Role conflict may have caused more distress than role change, primarily because consistency of behavior is a valuable attribute of a good doctor. Role conflicts were somewhat more likely to produce large changes than role change.

New learning was less common in this area of change than in the study as a whole, partly because very few formal educational programs are directed to the personal lives of physicians.

When the physicians undertook learning something about their families or community roles, they were more likely to concentrate on specific problems and choose deliberative approaches. In the context of the broad understandings they had of family and community life, they used learning to identify and weigh the alternatives open to them regarding specific issues or problems. In making more dramatic changes, such as role abandonment and role redefinitions, they were more likely to resort to informal learning resources and strategies, or in other words, turn to others in their social milieus rather than books or courses. This same tendency would probably be observed in any general sample of adults. Nevertheless, it is clear that many of the physicians did not know who to ask or where to get help.

Implications

Much of the learning needed to make decisions is secured early in life. A doctor's behavior in the context of family and community is, like anyone's, formed in the setting in which he or she was raised and in the philosophy of life obtained from that environment. What doctors do not learn early in their lives is how to be doctors, and how to reconcile that role with others that are more often taken for granted. Our interviews illustrated the need for physicians to bring the responsibilities of medical practice, family, and community into focus. It often appeared that doctors, confronted with conflicting role requirements, assigned priority to one set or another rather than attempting to reconcile them. For many, the area of higher priority was the family. Changes were made in clinical practice in order to reconcile the differences between professional expectations and those perceived as appropriate to family members.

A stock image of the physician, one that is often supported by medical training, is of someone who practices "hard ball" medicine, who is capable of putting everything except patient care on hold. The stories told by physicians we interviewed belie this stereotype. Influences and pressures from nonprofessional roles altered professional lives, just as professional demands altered personal lives. Recognizing the extent of this interaction would benefit future physicians.

Developing a sense of proportion in responding to the demands of medical practice and private life probably takes place during the formal socialization process that accompanies medical education. Medical educators should recognize their opportunity to help. Marriages and new children are common events among medical students. These events are critical points in the integration of medicine and family life. If the demands of school and family are balanced appropriately in these first tries, a pattern of life that maintains an appropriate balance may follow. If, on the other hand, a pattern develops in which one or the other of these dimensions is neglected, the opportunity to learn and adjust may be lost. In effect, family events of medical students may present medical educators with "teachable moments," junctures at which the right kind of help may prevent future dilemmas.

The right kind of help may take many forms. It may be that medical schools could provide family counseling services to help resolve conflicts and build coping skills. It may be feasible to establish support groups with trained leaders, to enable students, particularly women students (who face sizeable burdens in caring for children), to share and benefit from each other's experiences. It may be that written materials dealing directly with the problems of doctor and spouse, doctor and parent, and doctor and citizen may be useful ways to orient student physicians to multiple role expectations and role conflicts. Any of these actions could mediate the power of family and community relationships to generate changes in medical practice, and of medical practice to generate changes in family and community life.

Physicians currently in practice also need to address these problems. Professional associations, concerned both with physicians' well-being and with quality of care, would do well to investigate the influence of conflicting personal and professional roles on occurrences of malpractice and physicians' suicides, to take two examples. State and national professional associations already sponsor services for impaired physicians, many of whom attribute their problems to the stress of balancing practices with other roles. Preventive efforts focusing in these areas might have a high yield. The focus of research should neither neglect the influence of family and community roles on medical practice, nor focus on the negative aspects. Several of our subjects reported that their experiences as spouses or parents altered their practices in positive ways.

Women in medicine continue to deserve special attention in social and behavioral research. Many of the women in our sample expressed unhappiness as a result of mixing the roles of wife, mother, and physician. Anger, frustration, and disillusionment were often apparent, because mechanisms to support them in their various roles were not present. However, many women indicated that fellow physicians served as role models and mentors. Since it is likely that the number of female physicians will continue to increase over time (Heins 1985), formal efforts should be made by professional societies, medical schools, and hospitals to generate valid information and help with solutions.

Although nurturing and care of a family continues to rest largely on the shoulders of women (Robinson et al. 1987), the resulting conflicts should not be regarded as purely a woman's problem, and men should not be left out of the research or the solution. Some of the men in our sample made important contributions to their family lives and were markedly influenced by their family and community roles.

REFERENCES

Goffman, E. 1959. The presentation of self in everyday life. New York: Doubleday Anchor Books.

Heins, M. 1985. Update: Women in medicine. *Journal of the American Medical Women's Association* 40:43–50.

Rinke, C. M. 1981. The professional identities of women physicians. *Journal of the American Medical Association* 245:2419–2421.

Robinson, L., et al. 1987. Sex role stereotyping: Reactions of women anesthesiologists. *Journal of the American Medical Women's Association* 42:15–18.

12

A Theory of Learning and Change

Robert D. Fox,
Paul E. Mazmanian,
and R. Wayne Putnam

Without theory, research and practice are without form. Theory provides a skeleton of explanation and prediction that gives shape and structure to empirical investigations that, in turn, direct the practice of professions. It is not, however, immutable or even necessarily factual. At their best, theories are well-constructed, reality-based guesses about what happens, how, and why. Yet these highly credible guesses permit more tightly focused, hypothesis-based experiments, aimed at specific parts of the theory, to add or subtract support for its powers to explain and predict. The results of careful research and careful evaluation add the muscle and flesh to a theory, enabling it to guide those who study, teach, or practice.

Theories must be abstract because they must accommodate and organize an ever-changing body of facts. Part of the test of the quality of a theory is the array of changing facts that the explanations and predictions are able to encompass. Good general theories, such as those found in physics, have long histories of successful and unsuccessful challenges. When challenged successfully, theories have been rejected and replaced, or modified to accommodate new evidence or new ideas. In newer fields, such as education, theoretical foundations are embryonic. Such is the case in theories of change and learning in adulthood, where, as is noted by Merriam (1987, 197), "few of those [theories] reviewed have been empirically tested at all, and none is supported by a substantial body of research."

This closing chapter draws together concepts from physicians' natural histories of change and learning to develop propositions that suggest a general model of

162   Lives of Physicians

the process of change. Fundamentally, we propose a plausible, logical, and most importantly, empirically-based description of what changes, why, and how.

In developing our formal explanation, we have been careful to follow accepted recommendations and guidelines for inductive theory building. First, qualitative data on change and learning were collected. Second, categories of variation (variables) were described and related to one another. Third, these categorical variables were defined as concepts in order to encompass the range of variation. Finally, in this chapter, we will use models and propositions to explain and predict how one concept affects another. This process for developing theory "from the ground up" preserves the valuable "real-life" associations among the phases of the change process, but in the form of a theory of change and learning that can guide future investigations.

Because the explicit purpose of this investigation was to develop theory, not to test it, no post hoc tests of statistical significance were used. Support for concepts and propositions is drawn from descriptive statistics and individual narratives provided by physicians and reported in the preceding chapters.

We believe that the process by which a theory is constructed should be reflected in its presentation. Given that there were three essential questions guiding our investigations, our discussion of this theory flows from these questions to the concepts of forces (why change was initiated), types of changes (what kind of change was made), and learning patterns (how change occurred). Next, propositions are formulated that describe how types of changes are associated with different ways of learning and forces for change. These propositions are then organized and presented as formal explanations of three major types of changes. Throughout, propositions relating concepts to one another are formally stated as if they were generally true, to facilitate understanding and to foster future research designed to test their validity. In order to ease the burden of grappling with these abstractions, a drawing of the model of change and a summary of the overall process is used to close this section.

FORCES FOR CHANGE

Understanding what leads to the initiation of a process of changing is a complicated but vital first step to developing formal explanations and predictions about the process of change. As was discussed in chapter one, ten discreet forces that press for change were identified. These ten forces originate in personal, professional, or social dimensions of life. They do not act singularly in most cases, although one force usually seems to establish a more central and more powerful role than others. This primary force is supported, and sometimes opposed, by one or more other forces. For example, pressure from a family role conflict was, in some cases, a primary social force, a first cause of change. This pressure was usually augmented by desire for personal well-being (e.g., relief from personal distress). Although the personal distress was important, it was

Figure 12.1
The Interrelationships of Forces for Change

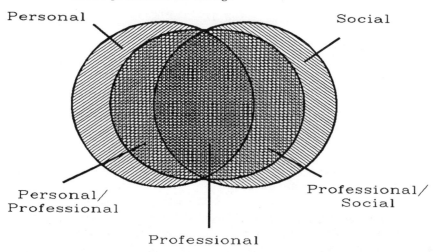

not primary but rather, secondary, and subsequent to the family conflict that caused change. Similar examples were obvious in many of the cases of change, but not all. Notably, desire for competency, a purely professional force for change, directly and singularly led to change in many cases. Figure 12.1 portrays the continuum of forces from intrinsically-generated personal forces to extrinsically-generated social forces for change.

The Venn diagram shows how personal, professional, and social forces overlap to describe a continuum of pressures for change. Although these forces for change arose from different dimensions of life, all were interpreted as personally important by our subjects early in the change process. For example, a request initiated by colleagues in medical institutions, a mixed professional and social force, has no power to bring about change unless it is interpreted as important to the individual. Although it is necessary to understand this linking of extrinsic events to internal drives, the primary force initiating the process of change affects both the path to change and the type of change that will occur. In the eyes of these physicians and, we suspect, in other professionals, these forces were the first and foremost causes of the drive to change. They had important consequences for what kind of change was to occur, and how it was accomplished.

DIMENSIONS OF LEARNING

Learning was usually a next step in the change process, but not always. In two-thirds of the cases described by physicians, learning was instrumental in changing the ways they practiced or the ways they lived. Whether or not learning activities were part of the process was related to the force for change. Learning strategies were most often associated with changes caused by purely professional forces (88 percent), followed by those forces with a personal dimension (e.g., personal, 68 percent and mixed personal and professional, 65 percent). Learning was least likely to be used in the change process when the force for change was more social—purely social (50 percent), or mixed professional and social (58 percent). The stories of change of these subjects affirm the tendency not to use learning in the change process when the pressure to change came from a social dimension of life or practice. For example, chapters eight and nine point out that when physicians expected to benefit personally or professionally, they were more likely to learn than when the benefit seemed to flow to a health care institution or professional association. The following proposition describes the relationship between forces for change and learning:

Professional forces and personal forces for change are more likely than social forces to lead to learning as a means for change.

Our subjects described learning by its: (1) purpose, (2) method, and (3) resources. Purpose of learning varies from problem-specific to conceptual. Problem-specific learning is directed toward finding the best steps to take to solve a concrete problem. The puzzle is well-defined in the mind of the learner, its dimensions and boundaries are clear, but its solution is obscure or unobtainable without learning. With conceptual purposes, on the other hand, the focus is on understanding, and creating better defined and more organized ideas and thoughts. Here, the intent of the learner is more to develop the intellect than to apply a solution to a specific problem.

Although problem-specific learning was slightly more likely to be in the purpose of learning for these physicians (59 percent versus 41 percent), this may or may not generally be true of other professionals, or of adults in other situations. Only further investigations can illuminate similarities and differences among these groups.

As described in the following propositions, learning purposes also varied according to what caused the change process to begin:

Problem-specific learning is more likely than conceptually-oriented learning to be associated with professional and social forces than with personal forces for change.

Conceptually-oriented purposes for learning are more likely than problem specific purposes to be associated with personal forces for change.

Many stories of change described how physicians felt a lack of clarity about the characteristics of both the forces for change and the kinds of changes being made. From these descriptions, we believe clarity describes how well both pressures to change and their outcomes are understood or foreseen by the learner. Evidence substantiating the value of clarity as an important concept for understanding the process of change often appears in stories of change, and was accompanied by expressions of anxiety or discomfort when little clarity about either cause or effect was expressed. The following proposition describes the relationship between clarity and learning purpose:

Learning was more likely to be directed toward solving concrete problems than broadening conceptual understanding, when the force for change or the effect of change was clear and unambiguous.

This proposition suggests that there is an internal process by which learners formulate an image of the cause and the effect of changing. This internal ideation reflects how much of what kind of pressure is felt, and how much and what kind of difference may result in their lives or practices. The nature of this internal image of cause and result of change affects their estimations of whether or not they need to learn and, if learning is necessary, how they should learn. Gleanings from stories of changes suggest that this internal process moderates the relationship between forces for change, learning, and changes.

Method of learning refers to the way in which resources and information were ordered, structured, and processed. If the ordering and structuring of resources fostered contemplation and consideration, methods were classed as deliberative. For example, a respondent may have sought information on the strengths and limitations of a new procedure or piece of equipment, and thus, read articles on each and discussed each with a consultant, weighing one against the other, in the abstract.

However, if learning resources and information were structured and ordered to enable direct experience in applying knowledge and skills, learning was experiential. For example, if the learner wanted to be able to interpret x-rays, he or she may have learned by practicing under supervision of a radiologist rather than by reading or listening to lectures. Thus, an essential difference between deliberative and experiential methods of learning is the extent to which the method emphasized thought over interaction. Overall, fifty-three percent of changes accomplished through learning were characterized by experiential methods and forty-seven percent involved deliberative methods. The following propositions describe the relationship between forces for change and methods of learning:

Learning associated with professional forces is more likely to be experiential than deliberative.

Learning associated with social forces is more likely to be deliberative than experiential.

Because the medical profession or any profession focuses on application of knowledge through practice, it is reasonable that learning should emphasize experience. However, it is also logical that because understanding is essential, deliberation is the primary method for learning in some of the cases. When others (in the workplace, home, or community) cause change, it requires more emphasis on consideration, probably because these kinds of pressures for change, and the changes they imply, are often vague. Clarifying cause and effect in these situations is essential to changing and learning. The narratives in the preceding chapters reinforce this proposition.

Resources were categorized according to two interrelated factors: Their importance and their legitimacy. Resources were identified by our subjects as primary, or most important. They were grouped according to the extent they were viewed as formally sanctioned for their value for learning, with those clearly sanctioned classed as formal and all others classed as informal. However, the classification was difficult and our confidence in the rightness of it is limited. Consequently, other than noting that formal resources were most often primary to learning overall, and that this was especially true when learning was associated with professional forces, no formal abstractions or propositions seem warranted. More controlled study of this important dimension is essential if its role in the process of change is to be understood.

TYPES OF CHANGES

The third set of concepts and propositions essential to understanding the process of change is tied to differences in the types of changes that resulted from pressures to change and the learning that often followed these pressures. As described in Chapter One, cases of change were assigned to four categories that described how changes varied from case to case. Although these different types of changes may indicate continual variation when considered overall, they are considered here as categories, with the expectation that future investigations may be more specific about their exact natures.

The first type of changes, accommodations, were small and simple changes often accompanied by negative reaction. They accounted for sixteen percent of all changes. A second type, adjustments, were generally larger changes that showed incremental differences in some element or aspects of lives or practices. These incremental changes accounted for almost two-thirds of all changes (62 percent). Redirections (18 percent of all changes) and transformations (4 percent of all changes) were larger and more complex changes in the structure of lives and practices, reflecting the addition, subtraction, or reorganization of major elements, such as adding or dropping major areas of practices, getting divorced and married, or relocating homes or practices. Together these structural changes accounted for twenty-two percent of all changes.

Each of these kinds of changes tended to be associated with different types of learning and forces for change in ways that made each predictable based on a set of interrelated propositions grounded in the data. In the following sections, incremental changes (adjustments in lives or practices), structural changes (the larger and more complex changes), and accommodations (small, simple acquiescence) are analyzed through interrelated propositions that explain and predict the roles of forces and learning in each type. It is at this point that the concepts and propositions are brought together to present a theory explaining more formally the process of change as it surfaced from our data. The theory is organized around each of three types of changes: *Incremental* changes, which were the most common of all types of changes in our subjects; *structural* changes, which included both redirections and transformations; and *accommodations*, which were the least common and smallest of the changes described by our subjects.

Incremental Changes

The following propositions are offered to explain how incremental changes are made.

Professional forces are more likely than other forces to lead to new learning activities.

As was noted earlier, new learning was associated with professional forces for change in eighty-eight percent of the cases of change caused by professional forces. Moreover, in change caused by desire for competence, new learning was present in ninety-two percent of the cases.

When learning is related to professional forces, it is more likely to be problem-specific than conceptual in purpose.

In sixty-five percent of the cases where professional forces led to learning, learning purpose was problem-specific.

When learning is related to professional forces, it is more likely to be experiential than deliberative.

Learning associated with professional forces was experiential in sixty-three percent of the cases. The pattern of learning in which learning was directed toward specific problems and experiential methods was present in almost forty-seven percent of the cases where professional forces led to change.

Learning is associated with most incremental changes.

In seventy-six percent of incremental changes, learning was characteristic of the change process.

Learning associated with incremental changes is more likely to be directed toward specific problems than conceptual understanding.

In sixty-one percent of incremental changes, learning was directed toward solving specific problems.

Learning associated with incremental changes is more likely to be experiential than deliberative.

Sixty-eight percent of all experiential learning led to incremental changes. In more than two of every three cases where an incremental change was the outcome, experiential methods of learning were utilized to make the change.

Professional forces for change and incremental changes are more likely to be understood clearly than other forces or types of changes.

Although this has been discussed earlier, it bears emphasis. Many years of medical training and experience clarify the nature of both professional forces for change and their consequences. Physicians often expressed that they "knew what had to be done" and "why."

The clearer the understanding of the force for change and its consequences, the more likely learning will be directed toward specific problems rather than broad conceptual understanding.

This was discussed earlier and is supported by the descriptions of change in preceding chapters. The essential logic is that learning in adulthood is a function of the need to develop understanding and to solve concrete problems. In some cases a clear understanding of problems is necessary to their solutions. In others, application flowed from understanding. Finally, in some cases, a richer understanding was the end point of the change process.
Therefore:

Professional forces are more likely than other forces to lead to learning characterized by problem specific purposes and experiential methods which lead to incremental changes.

Structural Changes

The explanation of structural changes follows a different path, leading back to personal as opposed to professional forces. The following propositions are offered to explain structural changes.

Personal forces for change are more likely than social forces to lead to learning.

This was true whenever a personal dimension of the force for change was present. Specifically, in sixty-eight percent of cases of change caused by personal forces and in sixty-five percent of cases of change caused by mixed personal and professional forces, learning was associated with changing.

Learning is usually associated with structural changes.

In eighty percent of redirections and eighty-two percent of transformations, learning was associated with changing. In 134 of the 167 cases of structural changes, physicians reported that they needed to learn in order to change. Most often, this learning was lengthy and complicated.

The nature of structural changes is less clearly understood before change is made than is the nature of accommodations or incremental changes.

This is a logical deduction, but it is also supported by physicians' expressions of ambiguity about making larger, more complex changes.

Lack of clarity is more likely to lead to conceptual rather than problem specific purposes.

This was discussed under incremental changes.
Therefore:

Personal forces are more likely to lead to new learning oriented toward conceptual understanding and to structural change.

Although personal forces played a role in only twenty-eight percent of all changes, they accounted for forty-three percent of all structural changes. In the majority of the cases where structural change was caused by personal forces, learning was conceptual.

Accommodations

Accommodations are a special class of small, simple changes. They differ from other classes because these changes are usually made with apathy, reluctance or anger. These are not the changes that are sought actively, rather they are acts of acquiesence. The following propositions describe the process of reaching accommodations. Each proposition contributes to overall links between forces and learning patterns.

Social forces are less likely than others to result in learning.

When mixed professional/social and purely social forces caused change, learning was present in only fifty-eight percent and fifty percent of the cases respectively. This is well below the extent to which learning was utilized as a means for making changes when personal or professional forces drove change.

Social forces are less likely than personal or professional forces to be clearly understood by those making changes.

This proposition was discussed earlier. Pressures from the environment are interpreted rather than generated from within. Therefore, social forces as initiators of the change process are less clear.

Accommodations are less likely than incremental or structural changes to be associated with learning.

Specifically, learning was associated with these changes in only forty percent of the cases. This may be compared to seventy-six percent of incremental changes and eighty percent of structural changes.

Accommodations are more likely to be associated with negative feelings.

Primary evidence is drawn from the stories of change forced by regulations, institutions, and organizations, discussed in chapters ten, nine, and eight respectively.
Therefore:

Social forces are less likely than other forces to lead to learning, but more likely to lead to smaller changes that are perceived negatively.

The Special Role of Clarity

Clarity denotes how well our subjects were able to define and describe the forces causing change, and imagine the consequences of making changes. Its primary effect was on the purpose of learning. Lack of clarity was most evident when social forces led to change or when one was contemplating a complex structural change. Because being unclear about why change is necessary, or what its consequences will be, means losing some control over the process of change, lack of clarity provokes anxiety. Thus, clarity may also be related to the disinterested or negative expressions often associated with accommodations, and changes characterized by compliance, usually with social pressures.

TO THE RESEARCH COMMUNITY

If you are disposed to believe the stories of change by physicians and the analyses of these stories, then the theory proposed must become an agenda for future research directed toward testing specific hypotheses and the measurement of variables. It is our belief that, even more effectively than the qualitative and descriptive analyses presented here, controlled scientific investigation will support these explanations and predictions. If you are disposed to doubt the veracity of this study, so much the better. Critical analysis and carefully constructed studies can only contribute to our understanding of change and learning in adults. Whether you tend to believe or tend to doubt, the study and the theory serve their purposes. They break the intellectual logjam that has characterized notions of learning in change for the past decade. They also promote a different scientific agenda for the future. Like you, we shall continue to work toward clear, useful, and most of all, valid ideas about change and learning.

A Model of Change and Learning with Implications for Educators

In order to facilitate understanding of change and learning, and to provide some of the implications for these propositions to those who educate professionals, it is helpful to have a visual representation of how the elements of the change process relate to one another. The figure below portrays the locations and connections among concepts that explain and predict change.

The change process begins with a force from one of five intrinsic to extrinsic dimensions. Forces may be: (1) personal, (2) mixed personal and professional, (3) professional, (4) mixed professional and social, and (5) social. These forces are perceived with more or less clarity. Among physicians, clarity of the force for change was greatest when it emerged as part of professional competence. Social forces, such as those emerging from relationships with colleagues, institutions, regulations, and family were perceived least clearly.

Educators of professionals should be aware that forces for change are critical determinants of how the professional will approach the learning situation and what kind of change he or she will anticipate. As motivations, forces may be profitably analyzed as part of the process of building a continuing education or staff development effort. For example, determining that the principal force for change is purely professional, as opposed to purely personal, suggests that experiential methods of education directed toward concrete problems likely will be more acceptable to learners than conceptually-oriented, deliberative methods.

It is also worthwhile to attempt to help professionals perceive more clearly what kinds of forces are prompting change. Our subjects did not always clearly understand why change was neccesary, especially when social forces were at work. In these cases, they were more likely to focus on gaining that understanding than on solving the concrete problems that they encountered in their lives or practices. One may be less concerned about the clarity of the force for change when it is principally professional, since our subjects seemed quick to grasp these reasons for making changes.

Forces are internalized to become important to professionals either through a longer building process or a shorter one involving a triggering event that dramatizes the need for change. Many times, triggering events occurred in close proximity to the force. Triggering events provide a window of high motivation to learn and change. It is vital to attend to these special opportunities, and to respond to them with appropriate educational activities. It may be that triggers for change can be simulated in the form of cases or natural histories (e.g., a bankruptcy, a failed procedure, or a family crisis) that enhance motivations without demanding that learners directly experience the event.

After the professional accepts that the force for change is important, a mental image of what kind of change is necessary develops. Like the nature of forces for change, this image may vary from clear to unclear. With the image of change in mind, the individual judges the extent to which he or she is able to make the

Figure 12.2
The Process of Change and Learning

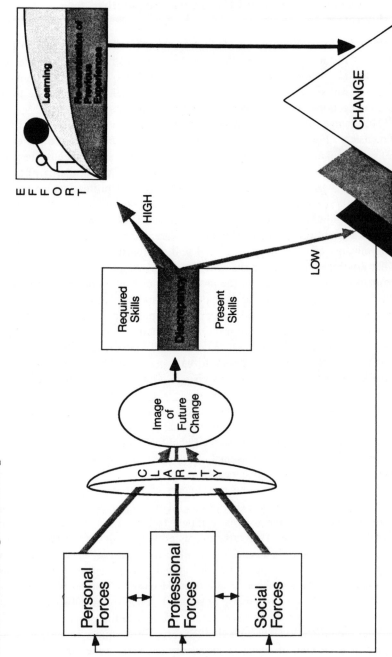

change, whether or not the present level of knowledge and skill is adequate compared to the level of knowledge and skill needed to make the change. If he or she believes his or her capabilities are sufficient, the change is made. If not, a plan for learning to develop capabilities to make the change is pursued.

Because the image of change, like the force for change, can be fuzzy, educators can facilitate the change process by being more clear about the specific changes that are promoted through their programs. Integrating information about the nature of a change promoted through an educational program allows the learner to focus more on specific problems that lie at the heart of the need for change. It also guarantees a kind of "informed" consent about what is likely to result from participation in education. Naturally, it would be best to develop the image of change endorsed by the program from information about the image of change held by learners.

Educators can also help learners to see what knowledge and which skills are essential for specific changes, and provide learners with ways to help them judge where they are in relationship to what is essential for making a change. In medicine, self-assessments are presently available, but they are more directed toward judging the adequacy of an overall store of knowledge in a specific area, rather than knowledge and skills associated with ability to change. As learners are better able to identify what they need to learn and focus on this, the efficiency, effectiveness, and pleasure associated with learning and changing is enhanced.

The strategies adopted for learning, including methods and resources used, are oriented to a purpose. Learning purposes range from problem-specific to conceptual. Purpose is affected by how clearly the force for change or the image of the anticipated change is understood in the mind of the individual. Learning to solve specific problems is associated with a clearer understanding of the cause of changing and the change, in all its potential effect. Learning intended to increase conceptual understanding is associated with less clear understanding of change. Also, conceptual purposes are more likely to be associated with personal forces for change.

Methods of learning refer to the ways resources are combined and used to achieve learning purposes. They range from deliberative to experiential. Deliberative methods emphasize thought over action while experiential methods foster interaction with people and things over contemplation. Deliberative methods are more likely to be associated with social forces for change than with other forces. Experiential methods are more likely to be associated with professional forces for change than other forces, and with incremental changes over other types of change.

Although learning resources varied from formal (perceived by the learner to be sanctioned by experts) to informal (not perceived as experts' opinions), the exact nature of this variation was less clear. Overall, learners showed a preference for formal resources in most cases of change.

The "natural" relationship between forces and learning patterns suggests a broader role for educators in helping to bring about changes in the practices of professionals. Many educators have seen their roles in change as limited to providing knowledge and skills, without paying very much attention to antecedents and consequences of change. Such a perspective may lead to programs that are not as obviously relevant to those who may be responding to many different forces or making many different kinds of changes. Frustrations over providing education to those who use such a program routinely versus those who do not—"preaching to the converted"—are commonly expressed. Our study supports that this concern may be warranted to the extent that participation in continuing education was often only a small part of learning associated with changing. Perhaps there are ways to make continuing education more effective in drawing in those who do not usually see it as an aid to the change process. For example, our study suggests that: (1) because a group of learners is responding to a variety of individual forces for change, multiple methods and purposes of education are warranted in most cases; (2) in certain cases, where social forces predominate (e.g., changes promoted through regulations, hospital policies, or peers), learning is less likely to occur unless issues such as competency or well-being are emphasized by educators; and (3) when learning is directed specifically to expressed wishes of learners to improve their professional competence or the capacity of their working environments, programs directed toward specific, concrete problems, that provide credible experience with new techniques, procedures, or information, are likely to be most acceptable to learners. This may be especially important when the planned change is relatively small.

Changes varied from small and simple to incremental, to large and structural. Accommodations, small, simple changes often perceived negatively, were associated with social forces and were least likely of the three to involve learning. Incremental changes were associated with professional forces and were most likely to be associated with learning. Moreover, when learning was associated with incremental changes, it tended to be problem-specific and experiential. Structural changes, redirections, and transformations of life or practice were associated with personal forces, and were likely to be associated with learning oriented toward conceptual purposes.

Many changes required of today's professionals are not small and simple. Our study suggests that the type of learning, and the precipitators of larger and more complex changes, are very different from learning and forces associated with incremental changes. When continuing education is offered as part of a strategy to encourage the adoption of major changes (e.g., career shifts such as geriatrics, sexual medicine, or preventive medicine), educators should consider learners' needs for: (1) a sense of personal commitment to the change, (2) a lengthy change process involving multiple experiences, (3) the opportunity to develop concepts that will undergird practices, and (4) the opportunity to deliberate over information instrumental to this new element in life or practice.

Learning sometimes played complementary roles related to the change process; it was used to help prepare to change, and to verify that the change was positive and valuable. The asterisks on the model indicate other places where the process of change was affected by learning.

These are only a few of the implications of our theory for the education of practicing professionals. The authors of the preceding chapters have followed their descriptions of the change process with other important implications and suggestions, developed out of these natural histories of change and learning in the lives of physicians. For all of these perspectives, the overall theme has been that there is more to facilitating change in professional practice than educational techniques. Facilitating change requires understanding and interraction of the educator with all phases of the change process. This global, as opposed to parochial perspective, will enable not only more effective and efficient, but also more ethical and enjoyable education and change. It is our hope that those concerned with the many changes made by professionals, which we view as the building blocks of progress, will examine our work with an eye toward generating ways to be more helpful to our clients and to the promise of progressive change.

REFERENCE

Merriam, S. B. 1987. Adult learning and theory building: A review. *Adult Education Quarterly* 37:187–198.

Appendix

Consent Form

To: The Physician Respondent:

        The Society of Medical College Directors
of Continuing Medical Education (SMCDCME) is
grateful to you for scheduling an interview. Over
100 North American Medical Schools are represented in
SMCDCME. Your participation as a respondent in this
research project may ultimately help medical schools
better respond to the learning needs of physicians.

Before any research may be conducted with human
subjects, respondents must be advised of the extent
of confidentiality, uses of the research, and
respondents' rights in regard to participating in the
project. The purpose of this project is to identify
changes that have occurred in physicians' lives or in
their medical practices and to describe how physicians
implement or respond to change.

The interviewer (signed below) represents SMCDCME. The
interviewer understands that you may discontinue your
participation in the interview at any time and at your
discretion. Please be advised that the data
acquired during this interview will be treated
confidentially. General descriptions may be included in
the interviewer's report. Specific identity will not be
reported.

Having reviewed this statement and agreed to participate
in the study, please sign as "Respondent".

_____   _____
Respondent   Interviewer

INTERVIEW GUIDE

1. Age of Respondent _____

2. Sex of Respondent _____

3. Majority of the practice is in an area with a population:

    A) _____Less than 20,000   B) _____ 20,000 - 50,000
    C) _____51,000 - 100,000   D) _____ More than 100,000

4. In general, how often do you talk with other physicians?

5. Majority of practice is:

    A) _____Institutional (e.g., a military physician or
            practicing in a state hospital)

    B) _____Non-Institutional (private practice)

    C) _____Does not Practice

6. Full-time Faculty of an Academic Health Science Center?

    A) _____Yes   B) _____No

7. Specialty/Subspecialty
    _____

8. What is the location and setting of the interview?
    _____

    _____

9. What changes have you made or have occurred in your
    medical practice or in your life within the past
    year?

    [Change may be thought of as a large or small
     alteration in what you do, how you do it, how you
     feel or all three.]

Follow-up question:

-- Can you be more specific about what exactly changed?

[At the point when the respondent cannot recall any changes, provide him/her the handout.]

10.   When did this change occur?

11.   What caused this change to occur?

>   Alternate phrasings: What led up to this change? How did this change come about?   Why did this change occur?
>
>   Follow-up questions:
>
>   -- What was the sequence of events that led to or caused this change?
>
>   -- How did you feel about these events?

12.   Did you seek information or attempt to develop your skills [in order to make this change] [because of this change]?

13.   What information or (skills) specifically?

14.   Did anyone help you develop your skills or gain this information?

15.   How much time, in hours, did you devote to acquiring information or developing your skills?

16.   In what order did you take these actions?

17.   Which resource was most important?   Why?

18.   What problems did you encounter in acquiring this information or developing your skills?

19.   Did these learning activities bring about changes other than the change we are discussing?

>   [Question 20, below, may have been answered in part by questions 12-19; in any case, confirm that answer.]

20. Did formal CME or other formal education play any role in learning associated with this change?

> Follow-up questions:
>
> --Was any formal instruction or instructional material used as sources of information or to help you develop your skills?
>
> --Did you attend programs, lectures or presentations, enroll in home study activities or self assessments, listen to tapes or other activities?

21. Will you estimate the number of hours of learning in regard to this change that was devoted to learning from educational materials or formal programs or presentations?

22. When did you begin to seek information or to develop your skills related to this change.

23. Could medical schools have helped with this process?

> Follow-up questions:
>
> --How could they have helped?
>
> --Why not? (to the response "No").

At about 45-50 minutes into the interview <u>or</u> at the point where no more changes can be recalled, ask the respondent -

> How do you use CME in your role as a physician?
>
> Does it ever relate to change?
>
> How?

Last Question:

In order to develop a long-term perspective on change, learning and education in medical practice we would like to return to you with either an additional interview or questionnaire once a year for the next five years. This follow-up will take no more than one hour of your time, and you may change your mind about participation at any time. Will you agree to participate?

Prompt Sheet 1

The following are areas of change that physicians have reported. Have you made or experienced changes in any of these areas over the last year?

A. Changes in your activities as a:

1. Manager

2. Educator

3. Researcher

4. Family Member

5. Community Member

6. Hospital Staff Member

7. Professional Societies

8. Board Member (agency)

9. Consultant

B. Changes in your feelings about:

1. Your medical practice

2. Your patients

3. Your future plans

4. Your retirement

5. Career goals

C. Changes in characteristics of your patient population

D. Changes related to aging

E. Clinical Changes

The following are examples of changes in clinical procedures other physicians have reported. The list may help you to remember changes you have made in the way you practice medicine. Have you made changes in terms of: interviewing/history taking, test ordering, prescribing, therapeutic protocol, surgical procedures, patient education procedures/counseling, follow-up, or case finding and screening procedures?

Selected Bibliography

Altman, M. 1986. In Allen, A. S., ed. 1986. *New options, new dilemmas*. Lexington, Mass.: Lexington Books.

American Medical Association. Board of Trustees. Initiative on quality of medical care and professional self regulation. Report QQ, adopted by House of Delegation, June 15–19, 1986. *Journal of the American Medical Association* 256(8):1036–7, August 22–29, 1986.

Association of American Medical Colleges. 1984. *Physicians for the twenty-first century, the GPEP Report*. Washington, D.C.: Association of American Medical Colleges.

Barrows, H. S. 1983. Problem-based, self-directed learning. *Journal of the American Medical Association* 250:22.

Barrows, H. S., and P. Tamblyn. 1980. *Problem-based learning: An approach to medical education*. New York: Springer-Verlag.

Beeler, K. D. 1979. How to design and conduct self-directed learning: An essential goal in education. *Kappa Delta Pi Record*, October.

———. 1979. Student self-directed learning: An essential goal in education. *Kappa Delta Pi Record*, October.

Bell, D. F., and D. L. Bell. 1983. Harmonizing self-directed and teacher directed approaches to learning. *Nurse Educator* 8:Spring.

Bennis, W., K. Benne, and R. Chin. 1985. *The Planning of Change*. 4th ed. New York: Holt, Rinehart, and Winston.

Bertram, D. A., and P. A. Brooks-Bertram. 1971. The evaluation of continuing medical education: A literature review. *Health Education Monographs* 5:330–348.

Brookfield, S. D. 1984. *Adult learners, adult education and the community*. New York: Teachers College Press.

———. 1984. The contribution of Eduard Lindeman to the development of theory and philosophy in adult education: A philosophical discussion. *Adult Education Quarterly* 34(4):185–196.

Buchholz, L. M. 1979. Computer-assisted instruction for the self-directed professional learner. *Journal of Continuing Education in Nursing* 10(1):12–14.

Cervero, R. M. 1988. *Effective continuing education for professionals*. San Francisco: Jossey-Bass.

Cervero, R. M., and K. H. Dimmock. 1987. A factor analytic test of Houle's typology of professionals' models of learning. *Adult Education Quarterly* 37:125–129.

Chene, A. 1983. The concept of autonomy in adult education: A philosophical discussion. *Adult Education Quarterly* 34(1):38–47.

Chin, R., and K. D. Benne. 1976. General strategies for effecting changes in human systems. In Bennis, W. G., et al. *The planning of change*. 3d ed. New York: Holt, Rinehart, and Winston.

Cohn, R. E. 1986. The medical director—the untapped potential of the position. *Hospital and Health Services Administration* 31(6):51–61.

Coleman, J. S., E. Katz, and H. Menzel. 1966. *Medical Innovations—A Diffusive Study*. Indianapolis: Bobbs Merrill.

Covell, D. G., G. C. Uman, and P. R. Manning. 1985. Information needs in office practice: Are they being met? *Annals of Internal Medicine* 103:596–99.

Cross, P. K. 1981. *Adults as learners*. San Francisco: Jossey-Bass.

Davis, D., et al. 1984. The impact of CME: A methodological review of continuing medical education literature. *Evaluation and the Health Professions* 7:251–283.

De Bono, E. 1985. *De Bono's thinking course*. London: Ariel Books, British Broadcasting Corp.

Denson, T. A., and P. R. Manning. 1982. Current problems in medical practice as viewed by California physicians. *Western Journal of Medicine* 136:369–372.

Dubin, S. S., and M. Okun. 1973. Implications of learning theories for adult instruction. *Adult Education* 24(1):3–19.

Dunn, E. V., et al. 1988. Study relation of continuing medical education to quality of family physicians' care. *Journal of Medical Education* 63:775–784.

Erikson, E. H. 1963. Childhood and society. 2nd ed. New York: W. W. Norton & Co.

Finestone, A. J., et al. 1986. A practice integrated learning sequence (PILS). *Mobius* 6(1):1–5.

Fox, R. D. 1983. Discrepancy analysis of continuing medical education: A conceptual model. *Mobius* 3:37–44.

Fuchs, V. R. 1988. Perspectives: United States. *Health Affairs* 7(5):25–30.

Geertsma, R. H., et al. 1982. How physicians view the process of change in their practice behavior. *Journal of Medical Education* 57:752–768.

Georgopoulos, B. S., and F. C. Mann. 1962. *The community general hospital*. New York: Macmillan.

Gibbons, M., et al. 1980. Toward a theory of self-directed learning: A study of experts without formal training. *Journal of Humanistic Psychology* 20(2):41–56.

Goffman, E. 1959. The presentation of self in everyday life. New York: Doubleday Anchor Books.

Goldfinger, S. E. 1982. Continuing medical education: The case for contamination. *New England Journal of Medicine* 306:540–541.

Gould, R. L. 1972. The phases of adult life: A study in developmental psychology. *The American Journal of Psychiatry* 129(5):521–531.

Green, J. S., et al., eds. 1984. *Continuing education for the health professions: Devel-*

oping, managing, and evaluating programs for maximum impact on patient care. San Francisco: Jossey-Bass.

Harrison, R. 1978. How to design and conduct self-directed learning experiences. *Group and Organization Studies* 3(2):149–167.

Harvill, L. M. 1981. Anticipatory socialization of medical students. *Journal of Medical Education* 56:431–433.

Havighurst, R. J. 1973. History of developmental psychology: Socialization and personality development through the life span. In Baltes, P. B. and W. K. Schaie, eds. *Life span developmental psychology.* New York: Academic Press.

Haynes, R. B., et al. 1984. A critical reappraisal of the efficacy of continuing medical education. *Journal of the American Medical Association* 251:61–64.

Heins, M. 1985. Update: Women in medicine. *Journal of the American Medical Women's Association* 40:43–50.

Hiss, R. G., et al. 1979. Development and evaluation of a community-based pulmonary education system. *Proceedings of the 18th Annual Conference Research in Medical Education,* Washington, D.C.: November 1979:264–269.

Houle, C. O. 1961. *The inquiring mind.* Madison: The University of Wisconsin Press.

———. 1980. Continuing learning in the professions. San Francisco: Jossey-Bass.

Iglehart, J. K. 1986. Health policy report: Canada's health care system. *New England Journal of Medicine* 315:778–784.

Kerlinger, F. 1973. *Foundations of behavioral research.* New York: Holt, Rinehart, and Winston.

Kidd, J. R. 1976. *How Adults Learn.* New York: Association Press.

Knowles, J. H. 1963. The balance of biology of the teaching hospital. *New England Journal of Medicine* 269:401–406, 450–455.

Knowles, M. S. 1975. *Self-directed learning: A guide for learners and teachers.* New York: Association Press.

———. 1978. *The adult learner: A neglected species.* Houston, TX: Gulf Publishing Co.

———. 1980. *The modern practice of adult education.* Chicago: Follett Press.

Knox, A. B. 1977. *Adult development and learning: A handbook on individual growth and competence in the adult years for education in the helping professions.* San Francisco: Jossey-Bass.

Kolb, D. A. 1976. *Learning style inventory technical manual.* Boston: McBee and Company.

Kralewski, J. E., L. Pitt, and D. Shatin. 1985. Structural characterizations of medical group practices. *Administrative Science Quarterly* 30:34–45.

Lanzilotti, S. S., et al. The practice integrated learning sequence: Linking education with the practice of medicine. *Adult Education Quarterly* 37(1):38–47.

Levinson, D. J., et al. 1978. *The seasons of a man's life.* New York: Alfred A. Knopf.

Lewin, K. 1951. *Field theory in social science.* New York: Harper and Row.

———. 1975. Behavior and development as a function of the total situation. In Cartwright, D., ed. *Field theory in social science.* Westport, Conn.: Greenwood Press.

Lloyd, J. S, and S. Abrahamson. 1979. The effectiveness of continuing medical education: A review of the evidence. *Evaluation and the Health Professions* 2:251–280.

Manning, P. R., and L. DeBakey. 1988. *Medicine: Preserving the passion.* New York: Springer-Verlag.

Merriam, S. B. 1987. Adult learning and theory building: A review. *Adult Education Quarterly* 37:187–198.

Mezirow, J. 1981. A critical theory of adult learning and education. *Adult Education* 32:3–24.

Morris, W. 1976. The information influential physician: The knowledge flow process among medical practitioners. Ph.D. diss. Ann Arbor: University of Michigan.

Morrisey, M. A., and D. C Brooks. 1985. Physician influence in hospitals: An update. *Hospital* (September):86–89.

Moss, A. B., et al. 1966. *Hospital policy decisions: Process and action.* New York: G. P. Putnam's Sons.

Neugarten, B. L., and Associates, eds. 1964. *Personality in middle and late life.* New York: Atherton Press.

Nowlen, P. M. 1988. *A new approach to continuing education for business and the professions.* New York: Macmillan.

Perkins, D. 1986. *Knowledge as design.* Hillsdale, N.J.: Lawrence Erlbaum Associates.

Pfeiffer, R. J. 1983. Early-adult development in the medical student. *Mayo Clinic Proceedings* 58:127–134.

Richards, R. K., and R. M. Cohen. 1980. Why physicians attend traditional CME programs. *Journal of Medical Education*, 55:479–485.

Rinke, C. M. 1981. The professional identities of women physicians. *Journal of the American Medical Association* 245:2419–2421.

Robinson, L., et al. 1987. Sex role stereotyping: Reactions of women anesthesiologists. *Journal of the American Medical Women's Association* 42:15–18.

Rogers, E. M. 1983. *Diffusion of innovations.* 3d ed. New York: The Free Press.

Ruelas, E., and P. Leatt. 1985. The roles of physician executives in hospitals: A framework for management education. *Journal of Health Administration Education* Spring, 3 (2, pt. 1):151–169.

Schon, D. A. 1983. *The reflective practitioner.* New York: Basic Books.

———. 1987. *Educating the reflective practitioner.* San Francisco: Jossey-Bass.

Scobie, R. 1983. Situational teaching: Fostering self-direction in the classroom. *Curriculum Inquiry* 13(2):132–150.

Shortell, S. M. 1972. *A model of physician referral behavior: A test of exchange theory in medical practice.* Research Series 31, Chicago: Center for Health Administration Studies, University of Chicago.

Sibley, J. C., et al. 1982. A randomized trial of continuing medical education. *New England Journal of Medicine* 306:511–515.

Skager, R. 1979. Self-directed learning and schooling: Identifying pertinent theories and illustrative research. *International Review of Education.* Boston, Mass.: Unesco Institute for Education.

Stein, L. S. 1981. The effectiveness of continuing medical education: Eight research reports. *Journal of Medical Education* 56:103–110.

Sternberg, R. 1985. Critical thinking: Its nature, measurement and improvement. In Link, F. R., ed. *Essays on the intellect.* Alexandria, Vir.: Association for Supervision and Curriculum Development.

Stross, J. K., et al. 1983. Continuing education in Pulmonary disease for primary-care physicians. *American Review of Respiratory Diseases* 127:739–746.

Sweet, R. L. 1988. Pelvic inflammatory disease: Prevention and treatment. *Modern Medicine of Canada* 43:345–350.

Tarlov, A. R. 1986. HMO growth and physicians. *Health Affairs* 5(1):23–35.

Thomas, W. I., and D. W. Thomas. 1970. Situations defined as real are real in their consequences. In Stone, G., and H. Faberman, eds. 1970. *Social psychology through symbolic interactionism.* Waltham, Mass.: Xerox.

Tough, A. 1971. *The adult's learning projects.* Toronto: Ontario Institute for Studies in Evaluation. (6).

———. 1978. Major learning efforts: Recent research and future directions. *Adult Education* 28(4):250–263.

———. 1982. *Intentional Changes: A fresh approach to helping people change.* Chicago: Follett Publishing Co.

Vroom, V. H. 1964. *Work and motivation.* New York: Wiley.

Wergin, J. F., et al. 1988. CME and change in practice: An alternative perspective. *Journal of Continuing Education in the Health Professions* 8:147–159.

White, R. W. 1959. Motivation reconsidered. The concept of competence. *Psychological Review* 66(5):297–333.

Williams, J. I., A. M. Bryans, and D. A. Davis. 1981. The continuing medical education of physicians in Ontario: Practices, needs and problems. *Ontario Council on CME: Report.* Toronto: University of Toronto Press.

Williams, K. J., and P. R. Donnelly. 1982. *Medical care quality and the public trust.* Chicago: Pluribus Press.

Index

Participants

Gloria Allington, CNP
University of Miami

Gail Bank, Ph.D.
Wayne State University

Don Campbell, Ph.D.
University of Wisconsin at Stout

David A. Davis, M.D.
McMaster University

Marjorie S. Foutz, Ed.D.
University of Texas at San Antonio

Peter O. Fried, M.D.
Rush Medical College

Martyn O. Hotvedt, Ph.D.
University of Texas Medical Branch at Galveston

Guy Jordon, M.D.
McGill University

Jocelyn M. Lockyer, M.H.A.
University of Calgary

Charles E. Osborne, Ed.D.
Southern Illinois University

Robert Anderson, M.D.
University of Arizona

Nancy Bennett, Ph.D.
Harvard University Medical School

Richard M. Caplan, M.D.
University of Iowa

Ruth Feryok, M.S.
University of California at Davis

Robert D. Fox, Ed.D.
University of Oklahoma

Harry A. Gallis, M.D.
Duke University Medical School

Patricia S. Iverson, M.P.A.
University of Oregon

Salvatore Lanzilotti, Ed.D.
Temple University

Paul E. Mazmanian, Ph.D.
Medical College of Virginia

John Parboosingh, M.D.
University of Calgary

Jacqueline N. Parochka, Ed.
University of Illinois at Chicago

R. Wayne Putnam, M.D.
Dalhousie University

Lucie Vogel, M.A.
University of Virginia

Harold A. Paul, M.D.
Rush Medical College

John W. Vester, M.D.
University of Cincinnati

Dennis K. Wentz, M.D.
Vanderbilt University

ABOUT THE EDITORS

ROBERT D. FOX is Professor of Higher Education and Research Associate in the Research Center for Continuing Professional and Higher Education of the University of Oklahoma. His current research interests include adult development, learning, and motivation.

PAUL E. MAZMANIAN is Associate Professor of Preventive Medicine and Director of Continuing Education in Medicine and Allied Health at the Medical College of Virginia/Virginia Commonwealth University. The organization of continuing professional education, commitment to change, and contract learning are his current research interests.

R. WAYNE PUTNAM is Assistant Dean for Continuing Medical Education at Dalhousie University, Halifax, Nova Scotia. His special interests are community hospital-based programs and evaluation of the effectiveness of education in the area of health promotion.